The Processing Program

Level 1

2nd Edition

Using Language Webs and Altered Auditory Input to Improve Comprehension

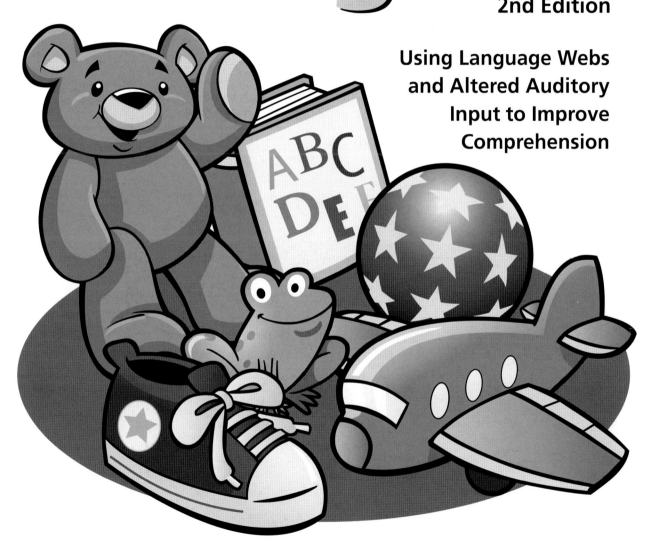

by Sandra McKinnis
Edited by Amber Hodgson • Illustrated by Chuck Hart

Super Duper® Publications • Greenville, South Carolina

© 2000 by Thinking Publications®
© 2008, 2012 by Super Duper® Publications

Super Duper® Publications grants limited rights to individual professionals to reproduce and distribute pages that indicate duplication is permissible. Pages can be used for student instruction only and must include Super Duper® Publications' copyright notice. All rights are reserved for pages without the permission-to-reprint notice. No part of these pages may be reproduced in any form, electronic or mechanical, including photocopy, recording, or any information storage and retrieval system, without permission in writing from the publisher.

09   08   07   06   05   04   03   02   10   9   8   7   6   5   4   3   2

Library of Congress Cataloging-in-Publication Data

McKinnis, Sandra, date.
   The processing program : using language webs and altered auditory input to improve comprehension / Sandra McKinnis.
      p.   cm.
   Includes bibliographical references.
   Contents: [v. 1] Level 1 — [v. 2] Levels 2 and 3.
   ISBN 978-1-60723-030-4 (v. 1 : pbk.) — ISBN 978-1-60723-032-8 (v. 2 : pbk.)
     1. Speech therapy for children. 2. Language disorders in children—Treatment.
3. Communicative disorders in children—Treatment. 4. Vocabulary—Study and teaching. I. Title.
LB3454 . M398 2000
371.91'4—dc21

                                                                                                                         00-021012

Printed in the United States of America

Cover design and Illustrations by Chuck Hart

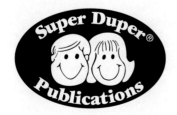

P. O. Box 24997, Greenville, SC 29616-2497 USA
www.superduperinc.com
1-800-277-8737 • Fax 1-800-978-7379

DEDICATION

This program is dedicated to my patients and their families who have taught me so much.

IN MEMORIUM

In memory of Nancy McKinley, Founder of Thinking Publications®

Contents

Preface vii

Acknowledgements.. x

The Processing Program–Level 1

Overview.. 3

Components 4

Language Processing and Language Disorders................................. 10

Program Instructions... 14

Altered Auditory Input Technique.. 16

Progressing Through the Sublevels.. 21

Reinforcement.. 22

Monitoring Progress.. 22

Appendices

Appendix A: Summary of the AAI Technique Use........................... 27

Appendix B: Determining your Natural Speaking Rate 28

Appendix C: Home Practice Letter 29

Appendix D: Progress Sheet 30

Appendix E: Outcomes 32

References 34

Level 1 Language Webs

Sublevel 1: noun (5 plates).. 38

Sublevel 2: noun + noun (10 plates) 48

Sublevel 3: noun + noun + noun + noun (10 plates).............................. 68

Sublevel 4: noun + noun + noun—*first two the same* (4 plates) 88

Sublevel 5: noun + noun + noun—*first one the same* (4 plates) 96

Sublevel 6: noun + noun + noun—*all different* (4 plates)..................... 104

Sublevel 7: noun + singular/plural (8 plates) 112

Sublevel 8: noun + plural + noun (4 plates) 128

Sublevel 9: size + noun (2 plates) 136

Sublevel 10: (size + noun) + (size + noun) (4 plates) 140

#TPX-27701 *The Processing Program: Level 1–2nd Edition* • ©2012 Super Duper® Publications • www.superduperinc.com   v

The Processing Program

Sublevel 11 noun + (size + singular/plural) (4 plates) 148

Sublevel 12: noun + (size + singular/plural) + noun + (size + singular/plural) (4 plates).... 156

Sublevel 13: color + noun (4 plates) 164

Sublevel 14: (color + noun) + (color + noun) (4 plates) 172

Sublevel 15: (color + noun) + (color + singular/plural) (4 plates) 180

Sublevel 16: (color + singular/plural) + (color + singular/plural) (4 plates) 188

Sublevel 17: size + color + noun (3 plates) 196

Sublevel 18: noun + (size + color + singular/plural) (7 plates) 202

Sublevel 19: noun + (preposition + noun) (6 plates) 216

Sublevel 20: singular/plural + (preposition + noun) (6 plates) 228

Sublevel 21: (size + noun) + (preposition + noun) (6 plates) 240

Sublevel 22: (size + singular/plural) + (preposition + noun) (6 plates) 252

Sublevel 23: (size + color + noun) + (preposition + noun) (6 plates) 264

Sublevel 24: (size + color + singular/plural) + (preposition + noun) (6 plates) 276

Sublevel 25: quantity + size + singular/plural (3 plates) 288

Sublevel 26: noun + quantity + (color + noun) (6 plates) 294

Sublevel 27: noun + (quantity + size + noun) (2 plates) 306

Sublevel 28: noun + quantity + (size + singular/plural) (4 plates) 310

Sublevel 29: (+/- quantity + noun) + quantity + (size + color + singular/plural)
            (4 plates) 318

Sublevel 30: (+/- quantity + singular/plural) +/- quantity + (size + color + noun) +
            (preposition + pronoun (5 plates) 326

Sublevel 31: (+/- quantity + singular/plural) +/- (quantity +/- size + singular/plural) +/-
            (preposition + pronoun) (6 plates) 336

Sublevel 32: (+/- quantity + singular/plural) +/- (quantity +/- size +/- color
            + singular/plural) +/- (preposition + pronoun) (6 plates) 348

Preface

Welcome to *The Processing Program–Second Edition*. This new program is an update of the original program published in 2000 by Thinking Publications®. *The Processing Program–2nd Ed.* has additional vocabulary and concepts as well as new sublevels. Some of the original sublevels have been expanded and several new types of sublevels have been added.

The development of the language framework and the picture stimuli for the original *Processing Program* began in 1984 when I spent a year in a small town in the outback of Australia. I had lots of free time! I decided to spend part of my time pulling together, into one cohesive sequence, some of the activities that I had found useful in working with children with language processing problems. As new research in the auditory processing capabilities of children with language impairment emerged and my experience broadened, I added new activities and incorporated new strategies. What began as a simple attempt to assemble all of my "auditory processing" activities into one folder, resulted in *The Processing Program*.

I organized the activities in both *The Processing Program* and *The Processing Program–2nd Ed.* to meet the following requirements that I found to be important when working with children with difficulties processing language. First, the sequences progress hierarchically from very simple to more difficult language tasks and can be used with children having a range of language difficulties—from those having significant difficulty with language to those with subtle problems. The activities create a series of tasks to use throughout the course of therapy as children progress in their acquisition of language and academic success. Each sublevel in the program builds upon the teachings of the preceding sublevel. This provides continuity from activity to activity, similar to Porch's idea of working "at the fulcrum of the curve" (Porch, 1979). In the Porch treatment approach, an initial level of difficulty for a child at a particular point in time is determined, and then, by working in small increments, the child's ability to complete increasingly more difficult tasks is facilitated. To implement the Porch approach, I needed a way to create a lot of items and a way to link each level to subsequent levels. The number of sublevels within *The Processing Program* and *The Processing Program–2nd Ed.* allows for this.

Furthermore, the stimulus items all begin with the same word, and the sentence stimuli is structured so that most of the important information is chunked at the end of the input to accommodate children with difficulty "tuning in" quickly enough (slow rise time) and those with fluctuating attention (intermittent auditory imperception). The child's response is a simple pointing response, rather than an object manipulation activity. This initial work resulted in the majority of the pictures, concepts, and language sequence for what I called *Levels 1* and *2* of the *Language Webs*. *Level 3*, the upper extension of the program, was added when I worked with older, elementary school-age children.

The Processing Program

The development of the technique for altering speech input to the children to make the input easier to process and learn started when I learned about the concepts of response latency, slow rise time, and intermittent auditory imperception in a *Porch Index of Communicative Ability in Children* training in 1980. Dr. Porch felt that slowing of input was helpful for children with these auditory processing problems. Later that same year, I attended a workshop given by Dr. Paula Tallal in which she shared her research findings on the auditory difficulties she had identified in children she labeled as "dysphasic." In this workshop, Dr. Tallal stated that her findings seemed to indicate that children with language difficulties were slower in processing the formant changes in the consonant to vowel transition in words than normal language users. However, when the formant transitions were lengthened using computer generated speech, the dysphasic children performed as well as children with normal language ability. When asked, Dr. Tallal stated that she did not think that slowing natural speech to these children would help. Since that time, a number of researchers have found that children with language difficulties appear to have trouble processing input at normal conversational rates and do benefit from a slowed rate of presentation (Ellis Weismer & Hesketh, 1996; Ellis Weismer, 1997; Montgomery, Majimairaj, & Finney, 2010).

As a clinician, I was curious to see if changing my natural speech input *would* accommodate the processing problems I had learned children with language difficulties experience. So, I began altering my way of speaking to see what would happen. First, I experimented with varying the speed at which I spoke and found that slowing of input did help some of the children. I discovered however, that there wasn't a standard amount of slowing that worked for everyone—each child had a "best" rate that was unique. Next, I experimented with stressing some words when speaking to the child to see if that increased processing and comprehension. I discovered that it was the pattern of pausing that seemed to make a difference for some children, not the added stress on particular words within an utterance. Finally, I experimented with altering the prosodic features of my verbal input to determine if I could impact processing and comprehension and found that, for some children, I could. I shared these ideas with a colleague in 1990, and she tried using these three techniques with her patients and found that she was able to facilitate improved language processing in her patients as well. The combination of these three techniques into one forms what we call the *Altered Auditory Input* (AAI) technique (McKinnis & Thompson, 1999).

Subsequently, we both began using the AAI technique with the Language Webs activities in *The Processing Program* and found it became an even more powerful therapy tool. This combination resulted in children moving faster through the Language Webs and, in better carryover of the concepts learned, into other language contexts. Using the picture stimuli for the Language Webs, we were able to determine the length of input a child could process and, at the same time, determine how to deliver the information by altering the speed, pattern of pausing, and prosody (the AAI technique) to boost processing efficiency and learning. Knowing the length and complexity of input the child could process, and the correct AAI technique that made input easier for the child to process, made all our other therapy tasks more effective. We could then help the parents, teachers, and the child's other communication partners know how to speak, so the child could better process speech input and understand.

The current program uses both of the features of the original program—Language Webs and the AAI technique. The Language Webs that comprise *Levels 1, 2,* and *3* are a great way to teach 126 basic vocabulary concepts and improve a child's ability to process these concepts in longer and more complex contexts. You can use the AAI technique during the Language Webs and all other therapy activities, and you can teach the technique to each of the child's communication partners.

Over the years, I have had many children tell me that my "shape program" was one of the most valuable parts of the activities I used in their intervention program. Many parents report that the AAI technique was the most useful technique that I taught them. I hope you find using both the Language Webs and the AAI technique as beneficial for the children you are working with as I have found them to be.

Acknowledgments

It is impossible to acknowledge all of the children, parents, and clinicians who have made positive comments and constructive criticisms about the *The Processing Program* over the past 20 years. It would not have ended up in its present form without this input. I thank all of you.

I would like to thank Molly Thompson, my friend and colleague, for her willingness to try the Language Webs with her patients and for her suggestions for *The Processing Program–Second Edition: Levels 1, 2,* and *3.* Together we refined the Altered Auditory Input technique, which was added to the Language Webs, creating *The Processing Program.* Her input has been invaluable.

Special thanks to the Alaska Scottish Rite for giving the families they fund for services and me the luxury of time. Because of their funding support, I have been able to work with children from start to finish in their treatment. Hence I have been able to learn what continuum of treatment works quickest and most efficiently. The members of the Scottish Rite organization are the best!! Thank you!

I would like to acknowledge Chuck Hart at *Super Duper® Publications* for the wonderful artwork created for this program.

I also would like to thank *Super Duper® Publications* for giving me the opportunity to share my ideas and the *The Processing Program* with you.

Thanks to my daughter-in-law Nadezhda for her help in typing the commands and picture descriptions. Spasibo!

Introduction

to *The Processing Program–Second Edition*

Introduction

Overview

Welcome to *The Processing Program–Second Edition*—the newest version of *The Processing Program: Using Language Webs and Altered Auditory Input to Improve Comprehension* originally published by Thinking Publications® in 2000. This new version retains the elements that made the original an effective language remediation tool. In addition, there is new vocabulary and concepts, along with new sublevels.

The Processing Program–2nd Ed. is a set of picture-identification tasks designed to improve language-processing skills. The professional/parent/aide presents directions with carefully selected concepts to the child, and the child executes the directions by choosing the correct picture.

There are three levels in *The Processing Program–2nd Ed.*: *Level 1* targets 46 concepts for children ages 3 to 6 years, while *Level 2* targets 101 advanced concepts for children ages 6 to 9 years, and *Level 3* uses many of the same concepts as *Level 2*, as well as 17 additional concepts, in longer and more complex command combinations for children ages 9 to 12 years. Age, however, is not the sole determinant for level use. For example, older children with more severe language disorders who need remediation of primary level concepts will still benefit from *Level 1* activities. The program features *Language Webs*, organized by linguistic concepts, and the Altered Auditory Input (AAI) technique, used to present the Language Webs to the child.

In a Language Web, concepts are arranged within a framework and introduced incrementally within the program. After the introduction of new concepts, previously presented concepts combine to form longer and more complex commands (i.e., directions). These strategic combinations form a Language Web. Each level of *The Processing Program–2nd Ed.* has a unique Language Web.

The use of the Altered Auditory Input (AAI) technique can help modify the verbal presentation of the commands to the child. In the AAI technique, there is an alteration of input (i.e., the spoken command to the child) with respect to the speed of presentation, the pattern of pausing, and the use of prosody. You use this alteration of input while the child is learning new concepts. After the child's performance reaches 100% accuracy at a particular sublevel, there is a gradual fading of the AAI technique. Also, you can teach this technique to the child's communication partners for use outside the intervention setting to speed generalization and enhance language learning in other contexts.

Intended Users

The Processing Program–2nd Ed. is appropriate for children having difficulty processing or learning language. It is beneficial for children with mild, moderate, severe, or profound language disorders, such as those due to developmental delays; autism; language-learning disabilities; attention deficit disorder (with or without hyperactivity); language disorders; central auditory processing disorders; head injury; hearing loss; cerebral palsy; and fragile X syndrome or Down syndrome. It can also be particularly helpful for children with cochlear implants.

#TPX-27701 *The Processing Program: Level 1–2nd Edition* • ©2012 Super Duper® Publications • www.superduperinc.com

The Processing Program

Speech-language pathologists, speech-language paraprofessionals, learning disabilities specialists, special education teachers, teachers of children with emotional disorders, and parents can use the Language Webs and AAI technique. These individuals may use *The Processing Program–2nd Ed.* with children individually because the AAI technique for each child is unique. However, you may use the program with small groups of children (e.g., two to three) if the children have similar needs.

Goals

The goals of *The Processing Program–2nd Ed.*, are to:

- Facilitate processing of various linguistic concepts, including nouns, prepositions, adjectives, and the singular/plural noun inflection / s, z, ɪz / (see **Tables 1–6**, on pages 6–8, for a complete listing of concepts).

- Facilitate processing of linguistic concepts in increasingly longer and more complex sentences.

- Help children achieve success in following auditory directions.

- Provide a technique to improve processing speed and efficiency, which can also be used in other intervention activities.

- Provide communication partners, including families and teachers, with a technique to help the child learn outside the intervention setting: in the classroom, at play, while someone reads to the child, in conversation with the child, and in structured listening tasks.

- Provide a link from oral to written literacy by using written language to help in the intervention process.

Components

The components of *The Processing Program–2nd Ed.* include the *Introduction* (which describes the Language Web frameworks and the AAI technique) and the picture plates with commands. In addition, there are suggestions for monitoring progress and involving other communication partners in the intervention process.

Language Webs

The Language Webs form the underlying organizational structure of the commands in *The Processing Program–2nd Ed.* by combining the linguistic concepts included in the program into increasingly longer and more complex commands. A framework of commands with a great deal of language redundancy is the result. Although each level of *The Processing Program–2nd Ed.* has a unique Language Web, the

4   #TPX-27701 *The Processing Program: Level 1–2nd Edition* • ©2012 Super Duper® Publications • www.superduperinc.com

Introduction

Language Web from one level frames the activities for the next level. This maintains continuity from level to level within the program.

Within each of the three Language Webs in *The Processing Program–2nd Ed.*, each new combination of concepts is a *sublevel*. *Level 1* includes 32 sublevels, *Level 2* includes 25 sublevels, and *Level 3* includes 14 sublevels. **Tables 1**, **3**, and **5** describe the Language Webs and the sublevels for *Levels 1, 2,* and *3*. As seen in these tables, the presentation of concepts appears first in simple contexts and then in various combinations with other concepts. This presentation provides incremental steps and repetition for processing commands of increasing length and complexity. **Tables 2**, **4**, and **6** present the vocabulary terms used to represent the concepts at each of the three levels.

Altered Auditory Input (AAI) Technique

In the AAI technique, the clinician alters the oral input to the child with respect to the speed of presentation, the pattern of pausing, and the use of prosody. The clinician then matches these modifications to the child's processing level. The combination of parameters needing altering in the AAI technique is unique to each child. Some children need only a slightly slower-than-normal speaking rate to better process what they hear. Others need a significant slowing of input. For other children, it is a requirement to slow the speaking rate and add pauses. Fewer children require an increase or decrease in the prosodic patterns of speech while some children require altering of all three parameters to process the spoken message.

The purpose for using the AAI technique is to make the spoken message (i.e., the oral input) easier for the child to process. This in turn makes it easier for the child to learn new language. The AAI technique strengthens language processing skills as well. When the child processes the new linguistic concepts with accuracy using the AAI technique, you can begin to fade its use. Fading the parameters of the AAI technique occurs by increasing the speed of input, decreasing pausing, and returning prosody to normal. For some children, elimination of the AAI technique can occur gradually. For others, parameters of the AAI technique may change over time as language learning and processing improve, but the need for some modification of the spoken message remains. This is particularly true for children with autism or other severe language disorders.

The picture plates and commands in *The Processing Program–2nd Ed.* help determine the parameters of the AAI technique to modify. The modification(s) used during the activities of *The Processing Program–2nd Ed.*, as well as during other intervention activities, maximize the benefits from all instructions provided. Ideally, the child's communication partners learn this technique in order to provide many opportunities during the course of everyday home, community, and school activities to improve language processing and, therefore, boost language acquisition. The AAI technique forms bridges among home, school, community, and the intervention setting, which increases generalization.

— The Processing Program —

| Table 1 | Language Webs | Level 1 |

Sublevel	Concepts
1	noun
2	noun + noun
3	noun + noun + noun + noun
4	noun + noun + noun – *first two the same*
5	noun + noun + noun – *first one the same*
6	noun + noun + noun – *all different*
7	noun + singular/plural
8	noun + plural + noun
9	size + noun
10	(size + noun) + (size + noun)
11	noun + (size + singular/plural)
12	noun + (size + singular/plural) + noun + (size + singular/plural)
13	color + noun
14	(color + noun) + (color + noun)
15	(color + noun) + (color + singular/plural)
16	(color + singular/plural) + (color + singular/plural)
17	size + color + noun
18	noun + (size + color + singular/plural)
19	noun + (preposition + noun)
20	singular/plural + (preposition + noun)
21	(size + noun) + (preposition + noun)
22	(size + singular/plural) + (preposition + noun)
23	(size + color + noun) + (preposition + noun)
24	(size + color + singular/plural) + (preposition + noun)
25	quantity + size + singular/plural
26	noun + quantity + (color + noun)
27	noun + (quantity + size + noun)
28	noun + quantity + (size + singular/plural)
29	(+/- quantity + noun) + quantity + (size + color + singular/plural)
30	(+/- quantity + singular/plural) +/- quantity + (size + color + noun) + (preposition + pronoun)
31	(+/- quantity + singular/plural) +/- (quantity +/- size + singular/plural) +/- (preposition + pronoun)
32	(+/- quantity + singular/plural) +/- (quantity +/- size +/- color + singular/plural) +/- (preposition + pronoun)

| Table 2 | **Sublevel Concepts and Vocabulary** |

Concept	Vocabulary
Noun/ Pronoun	airplane, ball, balloon, beads, bear, book, buttons, cat, cup, dog, dress, duck, frog, hat, it, mittens, mouse, ring, shoe, sled, sock, them
Singular/ Plural	/s, z, ɪz/
Adjectives	Size: big, little
	Color: blue, green, red, yellow
Quantity	a, a few, an, all, fewest, lots, most, no, one, only, some
Preposition	in, on, under
Conjunction	and, or, with

Introduction

Table 3 — **Language Webs** — **Level 2**

Sublevel	Concepts
1	noun
2	noun + noun
3	noun + noun + noun
4	size + noun
5	line + noun
6	color + noun
7	size + color + noun
8	(size/line + noun) + (size/line + noun)
9	(size + color + noun) + (size + color + noun)
10	(size + color + singular/plural) + (size + color + singular/plural)
*11	noun + (preposition + noun)—*above/below*
12	noun + (preposition + noun)—*beside/next to*
13	noun + (preposition + noun)
14	(color + noun) + (preposition + color + noun)
15	(size + color + noun) + (preposition + color + noun)
16	(size + color + noun) + (preposition + size + noun)
17	(size + color + noun) + (preposition + size + color + noun)
18	(temporal + size + color + noun) + (size + color + noun)
19	(size + noun) + (preposition + size + noun)
20	(+/- quantity +/- color + noun) +/- (preposition + noun) + (+/- quantity +/- color + nouns)
21	(+/- quantity + size + noun) + (preposition +/- size + noun) + (conditional +/- size +/- quantity +/- position + noun)
22	(+/- size +/- line +/- color + noun) + (preposition +/- size +/- line +/- color + noun) + (and/or) + (+/- size +/- line +/- color + noun)
23	(+/- temporal + color + noun) + (preposition + noun) + (temporal/conditional + color + noun)
24	(size + color + noun) + (preposition + noun) + (quantity +/- size +/- color + noun) +/- (conditional +/- size +/- color + noun)
25	combination of concepts

*Sublevels 11 through 18 use the nouns from *Level 1* to help introduce new concepts.

Table 4 — **Sublevel Concepts and Vocabulary**

Concept	Vocabulary
Noun	airplane, ball, balloon, beads, bear, book, buttons, cat, cup, dog, dress, duck, frog, hat, letter(s) [b, d, h, s, w, x], line(s) [diagonal, horizontal, vertical], mittens, mouse, number(s) [5, 6, 7, 8], one(s), ring, row, shapes(s) [circle, diamond, hexagon, rectangle, square, triangle], shoe, sled, sock
Singular/ Plural	/s, z, ɪz/
Adjectives	**Size:** big, biggest, large, little, long, longest, short, shortest, small, smallest **Color:** blue, brown, green, orange, purple, red **Line form:** thick (-lined), thin (-lined) **Position:** first, last, middle
Quantity	a, a couple, a few, an, all, four, least, most, none, one, some, three, two
Preposition	above, below, beside, next to
Conjunction	and, or, with
Temporal	after, at the same time as, before, first/then
Conditional	but not, don't/unless, except for, if, if/then, unless

The Processing Program

Table 5	Language Webs	Level 3

Sublevel	Concepts
1	(color + noun) + or + (color + noun)
2	(color + noun) + (temporal + color + noun)
3	(quantity + color + noun) + (quantity + color + noun)
4	(temporal + color + noun) + (temporal + color + noun) + (temporal + color + noun)
5	(conditional + size/color + noun) + (size/color + noun)
6	temporal + (size + color + noun) + (size + color + noun)
7	conditional/temporal + (+/- quantity +/- size +/- color + noun) + (+/- size +/- color +/- noun)
8	(+/- size +/- color + noun) + (in + positions + noun)
9	(+/- quantity +/- position +/- size +/- color + noun) + (preposition +/- sizes +/- colors +/- positions + nouns)
10	(+/- size +/- color + noun) + (preposition + positions + noun) + (+/- size +/- color + noun) + (preposition + positions + noun)
11	(quantity +/- color + noun) +/- (+/- conditional +/- quantity +/- color + noun)
12	temporal + (quantity +/- color + noun) + (quantity +/- color + noun)
13	combination of concepts
14	combination of concepts

Table 6	Sublevel Concepts and Vocabulary

Concept	Vocabulary
Noun	column, corner, letter(s) [b, d, h, s, w, x], line(s) [diagonal, horizontal, vertical], number(s) [5, 6, 7, 8], one(s), row, shape(s) [circle, diamond, hexagon, rectangle, square, triangle], thing(s)
Adjectives	Size: big, large, little, long, longest, short, shortest, small
	Color: blue, brown, green, orange, purple, red
	Position: fifth, first, fourth, last, left, lower, middle, right, second, third, upper
Quantity	a, a couple, a few, an, all, none, one, some, three, two
Preposition	above, below, beside, between, in, next to, to the left of, to the right of
Conjunction	and, or
Temporal	after, at the same time as, before, first/then/last
Conditional	but not, except for, if, if/then, instead of

#TPX-27701 *The Processing Program: Level 1–2nd Edition* • ©2012 Super Duper® Publications • www.superduperinc.com

Introduction

Picture Plates and Commands

Each level of *The Processing Program–2nd Ed.* includes a different set of picture plates and commands to use in the picture-identification tasks. *Level 1* includes 161 plates, *Level 2* includes 119 plates, and *Level 3* includes 65 plates. Each sublevel within a level has a different set of picture plates and commands. The number of picture plates per sublevel varies from two to ten. Generally, the first one or two plates in a sublevel review the concepts and vocabulary presented and thus tends to be easier.

Each picture plate has four to thirty illustrations. A list of commands accompanies each picture plate emphasizing the sublevel concept and concept combinations. The commands, printed on the back of the prior plate, are visible to the professional when the book is on a table.

The commands in each sublevel use vocabulary to represent the concepts (e.g., *cup, ball,* and *mouse* represent "noun"; *some, all,* and *only* represent "quantity"). **Table 2** (p. 6) lists the concepts in *Level 1* and the vocabulary (or morphological marker) chosen to represent the concepts. For most concepts, the vocabulary terms in *Level 1* appear again in *Level 2. Level 3* combines all of the concepts from *Levels 1* and *2,* as well as some additional concepts, into longer and more complex commands.

The vocabulary terms (1) are developmentally appropriate for each level, (2) can easily combine with other concepts to form longer and more complex commands, and (3) are typically difficult for children with language disorders to understand. Many of the terms were specifically chosen for their value in helping children follow oral and written directions in the classroom.

In addition to the concepts listed in **Table 2** (p. 6), you may use other familiar vocabulary terms within commands, with the assumption that children know them (e.g., *touch, and, with,* and *then*). Also, the concepts of quantity and singular/plural in *Level 1* are assumed knowledge in *Levels 2* and *3.*

On some plates, it is intentional to give the same direction with slightly different wording. For example, "Touch the duck below the shoe" and "Touch the duck above the mouse" will result in the same response. This helps children learn that there are various ways to state sentences while still maintaining the same underlying meaning. Also note that for commands including conditional concepts (e.g., *if...then*), the correct response may be to not respond, so the child needs to be given ample time to indicate no response.

Level 3 is an extension of the concepts taught in *Levels 1* and *2.* A set of written commands for *Level 3* is located at **www.superduperinc.com/processingprogram**. These commands can be printed, cut, and used with or instead of the spoken commands. Children can pair up and present commands to each other; one of the children can process and execute the commands while the other reads the commands.

The final two sublevels of *Level 3* present concepts that bridge to the academic setting (e.g., *between, instead of, fourth,* and *column,* etc.). These sublevels are generalization activities in which any

#TPX-27701 *The Processing Program: Level 1–2nd Edition* • ©2012 Super Duper® Publications • www.superduperinc.com

The Processing Program

number of concepts may be combined to form commands. You can use the commands provided in the activities, but many other possibilities exist. The last two sublevels can be culminating activities in which children generate commands for each other as well as process academically related concepts.

Language Processing and Language Disorders

Typically developing children between the ages of 1½ and 6 years learn to comprehend over 14,000 words just by listening to others speak (Templin, 1957, as cited in Rice, Buhr, & Nemeth, 1990). By the age of 4 or 5, typically developing children understand and use complex sentences that express the full range of communicative intents and their processing speed approaches adult levels (Montgomery & Evans, 2009).

It is incredible how effortless it is for children who are developing within normal expectations to break the code of the stream of auditory information that surrounds them to learn the language of their culture. A number of auditory processes contribute to the child's ability to accomplish this task, including such specific skills as auditory discrimination, localization of sound, auditory attention, auditory figure ground, auditory closure, auditory blending, auditory analysis, auditory association, phonological short term memory, working memory, and auditory sequential memory (Nicolosi, Harryman, & Kresheck, 1989). These auditory processes—the process of hearing; discriminating; assigning significance to; interpreting; and remembering spoken words, phrases, clauses, sentences, and discourse—form the basis for one's language processing ability (Nicolosi et al., 1989).

In contrast, the child having difficulty with language learning appears to have "glitches" in these basic inborn auditory capabilities. Not only is learning language through the auditory processes affected, but many of these children go on to have difficulty with reading, spelling, and writing, in part due to their difficulties in processing and storing language (Brady, 1997; Catts, 1997; Gillam, Cowan, & Marler, 1998; Shankweiler, Crain, Brady, & Macaruso, 1992; Montgomery, Magimairaj, & Finney, 2010, Studdert-Kennedy & Mody, 1995). Bourdreau and Constanza-Smith (2011) state that, "Children's working memory abilities at school entry have been shown to predict their overall academic attainment through adolescence." Alloway (2009) reports that working memory "serves as a better predictor of school success than IQ."

Causes

Researchers have posited a number of reasons for the language-processing problems some children experience. Temporal processing deficits (i.e., impairment in the speed of information processing) and limited cognitive and perceptual capacity have been suggested as causes (Ellis Weismer, 1996, 1997; Ellis Weismer & Hesketh, 1996; Just & Carpenter, 1992; Kamhi, Catts, & Davis, 1984; Merzenich et al., 1996; Robin, Tomblin, Kearney, & Hug, 1989; Tallal, 1975, 1976, 1990; Tallal et al., 1996; Tallal & Newcombe, 1978; Tallal & Piercy, 1973a, 1973b, 1974, 1975; Tallal, Stark, & Curtiss, 1976; Tallal, Stark, & Mellits,

Introduction

1985). The child's phonological short term memory and functional working memory are of particular importance (Boudreau & Constanza-Smith, 2011; Deevy & Leonard, 2004; Montgomery, 2002; Montgomery & Evans, 2009; Montgomery, Magimairaj, & Finney, 2010).

In examining temporal processing of children with language-learning disorders, all of the studies by Tallal and Tallal and her colleagues (beginning in the mid-1970s) and Merzenich et al. (1996) concluded that children with these disorders appeared to have more difficulty discriminating speech sounds at normal conversational rate, recalling the sequence of auditorily presented material, and processing the transition time of the first formant in syllables (i.e., the consonant leading to the vowel). When there was synthetic lengthening and presentation of the first formant of the syllable to the child using a computer, the performance (i.e., processing of information) of children with language disorders was comparable to that of their peers with normal language skills. Thus, the hypothesis of the authors was that "an auditory-specific and rate-specific perceptual impairment may be sufficient to explain the failure of dysphasic [language disordered] children to develop normal language proficiency at or near the expected age" (Tallal, 1976, p. 562).

A number of research studies by Montgomery et al. spanning 1999 to 2011 support the findings by Tallal and her associates that children with difficulty acquiring language have trouble with processing speed. Montgomery however adds that phonological short term memory and functional working memory play a role in the difficulties these children experience. Their studies have shown children with specific language impairment (SLI) to be poorer at processing and remembering one to three syllable nonsense words, in remembering new vocabulary, and in processing long versus short sentences.

Speed of temporal processing then may not entirely explain the language-processing deficits present in children with language delays. This difficulty with speed of processing may in fact be part of a generalized limited cognitive and perceptual capacity (Just & Carpenter, 1992). If it is true that children with language disorders have limited cognitive capacity, it would be useful to reduce the processing demands of language-learning tasks. One means of reducing the processing demand is to vary speaking rate. Ellis Weismer (1996, 1997) examined the effects of varying the speaking rate of linguistic models on the ability of children with language disorders to learn new lexical items. She concluded that fast speaking rates are detrimental to word learning. Although she did not find a "significant" effect to support slowing speaking rate for the group of children as a whole, some of the children with language disorders did benefit from a reduction in speaking rate; therefore, manipulations of speaking rate appear to impact some children's ability to learn new words.

Another alternative for modifying the processing demand of a language-learning task is to modify the prosody of the spoken message. Ellis Weismer (1997) and Ellis Weismer and Hesketh (1996, 1998) also examined the influence of prosodic adjustments on children's word learning in children with

#TPX-27701 *The Processing Program: Level 1–2nd Edition* • ©2012 Super Duper® Publications • www.superduperinc.com

The Processing Program

language disorders. They observed a significant effect for stress for production of new words but not for comprehension of the same words.

It should be noted that all the Ellis Weismer and Ellis Weismer and Hesketh studies differed from the Tallal, Tallal et al., and Merzenich et al. studies. Ellis Weismer and Hesketh used natural speech and complete words, phrases, and sentences in their studies. Tallal, Tallal et al., and Merzenich et al. used synthetically produced single syllables from a computer.

Recent research has supported these earlier findings and expanded our knowledge of the particular mechanisms that seem to interfere with these children's language learning ability. Studies carried out by Boudreau and Constanza-Smith (2011); Deevy and Leonard (2004); Montgomery (2002); Montgomery and Evans (2009); Montgomery, Magimairaj, and Finney (2010) revealed that children with SLI often have:

- Reduced functional working memory capacity resulting in more difficulty with longer sentences than shorter input.

- Reduced and inefficient phonological short term memory, especially for nonsense words, and presumably new vocabulary.

- A poorer ability to comprehend speech input at normal conversational rates, which may be part of a generalized slowing of processing across all modalities and/or a slower rate of cognitive processing.

- Trouble with simultaneous, multi-modality processing (i.e., having to process visual and auditory information while organizing a verbal response to the input).

Intervention

Altered Input

Traditional intervention activities for children having language-processing difficulties have included a wide variety of listening tasks requiring children to repeat series of words or digits, to follow auditory commands, or to answer questions. Two computer-based interventions purport to improve language processing; *Earobics®* (1997), developed by Cognitive Concepts, and *Fast ForWord®* (1998), developed by Scientific Learning Corporation. They contain computerized versions of some of the traditional auditory processing tasks for use with children. However, there are no recent research studies that find *Fast ForWord®* to be superior to clinician-directed activities (Gillam, Loeg, Hoffman, Bohman, Champlin, & Thibodeau, 2008).

Although *Earobics®* and *Fast ForWord®* have merits as remediation tools, intervention using these programs involves the child sitting at a computer for long periods of time listening to computer generated speech rather than engaging in face-to-face communication with others. An approach that modifies natural speech input to the child, such as the AAI technique in *The Processing Program—2nd*

Ed., has advantages over these computer-based programs. Modifying natural speech as part of a child's intervention program is easy to do at no additional cost to a family. You can use the modified input in face-to-face communication contexts, and you can teach it to all of the child's communication partners to facilitate language learning in other environments.

Ellis Weismer (1996) suggests altering a combination of variables, such as speaking rate, emphatic stress, and linguistic content, to maximize a child's language learning. This is exactly what the AAI technique employed in *The Processing Program–2nd Ed.* does. In using the AAI technique, the professional defines the modifications of the speed of presentation, the pattern of pausing, and the prosody of the spoken message input to maximize the child's language processing at the particular levels of linguistic complexity found in the Language Webs. The AAI technique makes learning the new concepts and linguistic combinations at the introduction of each sublevel easier.

Incremental Learning and Redundancy

The treatment philosophy that children learn best in incremental steps (Porch, 1979) and with redundant and multiple experiences over time (Ellis Weismer, 1997; Merzenich & Jenkins, 1995; Merzenich, Tallal, Peterson, Miller, & Jenkins, 1999) is the basis for the Language Webs as well as the idea that greater progress will occur if the focus of treatment is on improving the basic underlying language learning mechanisms rather than teaching a series of language tasks (Montgomery, 2002). Therefore, the focus in *The Processing Program –2nd Ed.*, is on teaching strategies for listening and comprehending within hierarchically arranged, developmentally sequenced, language learning tasks. The program builds functional working memory and phonological processing accuracy. The Porch concept of teaching "at the fulcrum of the curve" was a major consideration throughout the creation of *The Processing Program–2nd Ed.* In teaching at the fulcrum of the curve, you choose intervention tasks wherein the child is generally able to do the task at hand, but may exhibit a delay in response speed or have errors on up to 20% of the items given. The child practices this task until he or she completes it with no response delays or errors. The task then becomes slightly more difficult, and the child again practices to increase response speed and accuracy on the new task. In this way, by working in small, incremental steps, the child's overall skill level improves. And, as Porch (1979) states, the "processes involved in that task become available for all the more difficult tasks; therefore, all performance involving those processes improves" (p. 5).

Merzenich et al.'s (1999) neuropsychological and perceptual training studies have shown that humans are subject to powerful positive brain/plasticity learning effects throughout life, and there can be improvement of critical and basic listening skills at any age through intensive training. When multiple experiences of direct intensive training occur over time, there is a formation or strengthening of new neural groups and consequently a changing of the cortex. Further, Merzenich and Jenkins (1995) reason that intensive training that follows basic behavioral principles and increases processing requirements gradually, results in maximal reorganization of the neural mechanism.

The Processing Program

By teaching in incremental steps, professionals can also increase the automaticity of newly acquired language skills. In teaching new vocabulary and linguistic constructs, Ellis Weismer (1997) suggests that "new forms be introduced in highly familiar routines or scripts and embedded within a simplified linguistic context consisting of earlier acquired vocabulary and utterance construction" (p. 48). She further explains that there is accomplishment of automaticity through practice in repeated opportunities for meaningful use of forms and functions and by firmly establishing language skills before advancing to new goals.

The Processing Program–2nd Ed. contains enough items at each sublevel to facilitate "working at the fulcrum of the curve" as set forth by Porch (1979). Additionally, the Language Web frameworks within the program utilize incremental learning and redundancy. The Language Webs are not just a collection of auditory tasks that the child learns to do. Instead, each new sublevel in a Language Web is either a combination of prior levels or is the introduction of a new concept embedded within these combinations. Comments by Montgomery (2002) lend support to this idea in which he states that, "it might be useful, whenever possible, to link new words to words the child already knows" (p. 88). Thus redundancy in this program is a teaching strategy, and there is embedding of new concepts within prior language knowledge. This makes the new concept easier for the child to detect, process, and learn.

Program Instructions

The activities within *The Processing Program–2nd Ed.* are simple picture-identification tasks. The clinician presents a command (input) to the child, and the child then touches the corresponding picture to execute the command. *The Processing Program–2nd Ed.* can be the child's entire remediation program; however, it may be used in combination with other language-processing tasks and intervention activities.

Using *The Processing Program–2nd Ed.* for the first fifteen to twenty minutes of each session with the child is optimal. However, some older children who enjoy structured tasks can participate for longer time periods. As well, using *The Processing Program–2nd Ed.* at the beginning of each session with the child has a number of benefits. First, it is a wonderful warm-up activity that helps children "settle into" the session. Second, because children with language disorders have language-processing performance that may fluctuate from day to day, *The Processing Program–2nd Ed.* can help gauge how well the child is processing input on that day. This makes choosing additional intervention activities for that session easier. Having information about how a child is processing on a particular day is also valuable information to share with the child's family and teachers after the child's session. *The Processing Program–2nd Ed.* in this instance, functions as a "mini" diagnostic measure of the child's processing from session to session.

14   #TPX-27701 *The Processing Program: Level 1–2nd Edition* • ©2012 Super Duper® Publications • www.superduperinc.com

Introduction

Directions to the Child

It is helpful for children to understand why clinicians are asking them to complete the tasks in *The Processing Program–2nd Ed.* and why the auditory input is being altered. Read the following directions in blue to the child: I'm going to ask you to listen to what I say, and then you will point to some pictures in this book. Listen to the whole direction before you touch a picture. These activities will help you learn to listen and remember better.

For *Levels 2* and *3,* add this direction: Listen carefully, for a few of these directions you will be correct by not pointing at anything.

Then, explain the use of the AAI technique by saying: I'll talk slowly to help you do your best.

When you finish for the day, it is also helpful for older children to take a moment to reflect on how they feel about their performance including what modifications were helpful and what strategies they used to process the commands.

Determining the Beginning Level and Sublevel of Instruction

Before using *The Processing Program–2nd Ed.* with any child, you must first determine the beginning level (i.e., *Level 1, 2,* or *3*) of instruction and then determine the starting sublevel within that level. Determining the child's beginning level of instruction starts with an evaluation of the child's receptive and expressive language and language processing skills. You can administer standardized language tests during the initial assessment that yield a language-age equivalent. For example, children whose scores on receptive language tests are in the 6- to 9-year range begin at *Level 2* and those whose scores are in the 9- to 12-year range begin at *Level 3.*

Administering *The Token Test for Children II* (DiSimoni, 1978) is another way to determine the beginning level for a child. For example, if a child completes two- and three-element directions on Section 3 of *The Token Test for Children II,* and is functioning at the 4- to 5-year level on other language measures, begin with *Level 1* of *The Processing Program–2nd Ed.*

Once you determine the start level, do the following to determine at which sublevel to begin. Start with the first picture plate in Sublevel 1 of the beginning level and present the commands to the child at your normal conversational rate. Present the commands from the first plate of each subsequent sublevel. Calculate the child's percent of correct responses as you proceed. Typically, you calculate percent of correct responses after presentation of 10 commands within a sublevel. In some sublevels, commands may need repetition to derive 10 responses. Continue through the sublevels until the child's performance falls below 80%. The highest sublevel at which the child processes the commands at 80% accuracy is the beginning sublevel of instruction. For example, in the following scenario for *Level 1,* you would begin instruction at Sublevel 5.

#TPX-27701 *The Processing Program: Level 1–2nd Edition* • ©2012 Super Duper® Publications • www.superduperinc.com

The Processing Program

Sublevel	Concept	Child's response	% Correct
1	noun	+ + + + + + + + +	100
2	noun + noun	+ + + + + + + + +	100
3	noun + noun + noun + noun	+ - + + + + + + +	90
4	noun + noun + noun—*first two the same*	- + + + + + + + +	90
5	noun + noun + noun—*first one the same*	+ + + - + + + + -	80

Another way to determine the beginning sublevel is to note during informal tasks the length of input that the child processes. You can do this by presenting questions or commands of varying length and complexity, noting the child's responses, then choosing an appropriate sublevel.

Determining the Parameters of the Altered Auditory Input (AAI) Technique

After determining the beginning level and sublevel of instruction, determine the parameters of the AAI technique to modify. The parameters needing modification within the AAI technique are unique to each child. There is no standard amount of slowing, standard pattern of pausing, or standard prosody that works for everyone. For example, some children will increase performance when presented with sublevel items at a rate just slightly slower than your normal speaking rate. Other children will require significantly slower input. Typically, children with more profound language disabilities need the slowest rates. It is important to be aware that the requirement and amount of slowing or alteration of pausing and prosody may be more dramatic than you might think.

It should not be a concern that the child with language processing problems will perceive your alteration of input as strange or unusual. Children with whom you are using the AAI techniques may initially not comment on the modification but will when their language processing skills improve. This is important diagnostic information.

Besides the child's improvement in performance in the sublevel tasks, other behaviors will let you know that you are using the correct AAI technique. A typical response that occurs in children with use of the correct AAI technique is a calmer and more organized response to language input. Children typically will show fewer signs of frustration and sensory overload, such as inattention, crying, covering their ears, poor eye contact, echolalia, or refusal to complete language tasks. They also will attend to language input for longer periods of times. Along with increases in comprehension, children may also show an increase in expressive language. It is typical for the child to increase the number of syllables and mean length of utterance (MLU), to decrease the number of syllable deletions in words, and to show improvements in speech clarity with the

Introduction

correct use of AAI technique. This change typically occurs within the first few sessions with the child. Be sure to take the time to experiment in determining the correct AAI modifications for a particular child since it will make intervention more effective. Completion of this period of experimentation usually takes fifteen to thirty minutes of the first session with the child. The procedure for determining which parameter(s) to modify and to what degree is as follows:

1. Determine your own natural speaking rate. A typical speaking rate is generally in the range of four to five syllables per second. To obtain a gross estimate of your own speaking rate, use a stopwatch, clock, or watch with a second hand. Say a command at your normal speaking rate and note the time taken. Next, count the number of syllables in the command and divide the number of syllables by the time taken. Do this with at least five commands of different lengths, and calculate the average time taken. This is your speaking rate in syllables per second. Once you know your own natural speaking rate, you are ready to begin the process of determining the modifications to the AAI parameters that need to occur for a particular child.

2. Present commands at the selected beginning sublevel of instruction at a rate slower than your natural speaking rate, and note whether this increases the child's response accuracy. As you slow your rate, be sure to keep the pauses between words equal. You can slow your rate of speech by elongating the vowel(s) within a syllable, prolonging continuant sounds, or increasing pause length between syllables. There is no standard amount of slowing that works for every child, so use your natural speaking rate as a starting point, and slow that by two to three syllables per second. Some children require only slight slowing; others will need more. Speaking at a two- to three-syllable-per-second rate works best for most children. If the child responds to commands at the beginning sublevel with greater than 80% accuracy, you have identified the speaking rate (i.e., the speed of input) that works for the child. If not, you may need to slow down further or modify another parameter.

3. If slowing alone does not increase the child's percentage of correct responses, try slowing speaking rate *and* altering pattern of pausing. You may need to vary number of pauses depending on the length of the command. Typically, one to three inserted pauses are sufficient to improve a child's performance to 80% accuracy or better. Achievement at this response level establishes the appropriate combination of slowing and pausing. Note that slowing of input refers to the number of syllables you produce within a specific time period, while pausing refers to the insertion of silence at phrase boundaries. The following is an example of the same command presented with one to five pauses (• = *pause*). Remember that in addition to the pausing, each command is spoken slowly (i.e., two to three syllables per second).

#TPX-27701 *The Processing Program: Level 1–2nd Edition* • ©2012 Super Duper® Publications • www.superduperinc.com

The Processing Program

Number of Pauses	Command Presentation
One	Touch the truck • with frogs and a duck.
Two	Touch • the truck • with frogs and a duck.
Three	Touch • the truck • with • frogs and a duck.
Four	Touch • the truck • with • frogs • and a duck.
Five	Touch • the • truck • with • frogs • and a duck.

If the child's response performance improves, this is the correct AAI modification (i.e., slowing and pausing) to use.

4. If the child does not respond to the commands with at least 80% accuracy with a slowing of input and addition of pauses, try slowing, pausing, *and* increasing or reducing your prosody (i.e., the intonation and stress you use while speaking). Present items with either a monotone voice or a singsong prosodic pattern. Decreasing prosody (i.e., speaking in a monotone voice) is particularly effective with children who are autistic or with children who experience ADD, ADHD, or sensory integrative dysfunction. Increasing prosody (i.e., speaking in a singsong manner) helps children having generalized language delays, such as those exhibited by children with Down syndrome. Experiment with alteration of prosody while using the rate and pausing pattern that results in the highest level of accuracy to determine the most beneficial input for the child.

5. Once you determine and modify the AAI parameters that allow a child to respond with at least 80% accuracy, use the modification(s) as you begin within the sublevels. If, after working through steps 1 to 4, you still find that the child's performance at that sublevel does not improve, the child is most likely beginning at too difficult a sublevel. Back up to the next lower sublevel, and try steps 1 through 4 again. While this may be time-consuming for the first few children you attempt the AAI technique with, it does become much quicker with time (usually ten to fifteen minutes). After you determine the modifications of the AAI technique that increases processing for the child, you are ready to begin instruction.

Target Criterion

Use the AAI technique to increase the child's performance at a sublevel, and then ultimately fade its use. During the instructional phase of intervention, continue presenting commands for the beginning sublevel using the AAI technique until the child's performance reaches 100% accuracy. This may occur

Introduction

within one session, or it may take several sessions. Some commands may need repetition in order to reach this criterion level. When the child's performance reaches a 100% criterion level on a particular plate, begin fading the AAI technique. For example, in the following scenario, fading of the AAI technique begins at the third plate of Sublevel 4.

Level 1–Sublevel 4:

Plate	Child's Responses	% correct
1	+ - + + - + + + +	80
2	+ - + + + + + + +	90
3	+ + + + + + + + +	100

Fading Use of the AAI Technique

The goal when using the AAI technique is to increase the child's performance at a particular sublevel, and then fade its use at that sublevel. Fading use of the AAI technique is dependent on the child's performance. As mentioned earlier, when the child's performance reaches the 100% criterion level, fading of the AAI technique begins. The number of commands required to fade use of the AAI technique varies. Use the following sequence to fade use of the AAI technique at any particular sublevel.

1. If the AAI technique you use involves only slowing the rate of input, gradually increase your speaking rate in one-syllable-per-second increments when presenting the commands at the sublevel of instruction. You may be able to do this after only a few commands within a sublevel, or it may require the child to process many commands. Again, use the child's performance as your guide. When the child completes commands at a sublevel with 100% accuracy at a normal speaking rate, advance the child to the next sublevel within the Language Web.

2. If the AAI technique you use involves slowing the rate of input and altering pausing, first decrease the number of pauses, and then increase your speaking rate to normal. Again, this may happen within a few commands during one session, or it may take many commands over several sessions.

3. If the AAI technique you use involves slowing the rate of input, altering pausing, and modification of prosody, first return prosody to normal, then eliminate the pausing pattern, and finally return to your normal speaking rate.

When the AAI technique is no longer in use at a sublevel, the child is ready to move to the next sublevel. It is common for the parameter(s) needing modification in the AAI technique to change over the course of intervention. A child may initially need dramatic slowing of speech (input) and then

The Processing Program

later be able to process it at a faster speed. Or, a child may need frequent pauses in order to complete items at first and then later require none. Fewer children require alteration of the prosodic features, and most are able to process information with normal prosody after a few months of intervention. Again, you will need to experiment as you move the child through each Language Web. At each new sublevel, spend a few minutes experimenting with faster rates of presentation, different patterns of pausing, or modification of prosody as appropriate for a particular child.

Typically, the child needs the AAI technique for the first few months of instruction, and then he or she may no longer need it. However, other children will always perform better when there is an alteration of input, particularly when they are learning new information.

As a summary reminder of the AAI technique and procedure for fading its use, see the *Summary of AAI Technique Use* in Appendix A (p. 27). You can duplicate and laminate the summary, and keep it as a handy reference as you become comfortable using the technique.

Teaching Communication Partners the AAI Technique

There are two primary reasons for teaching the AAI technique to the child's communication partners. First, it allows the communication partners to decrease the number of communication breakdowns, and second, it maximizes the child's opportunities for language learning in naturalistic environments.

Communication breakdowns are common when adults attempt to talk with children with language processing problems. These children frequently respond incorrectly or inconsistently when spoken to, and adults may misinterpret these behaviors as defiance or a lack of cooperation.

Use of the AAI technique by the child's communication partners outside the intervention setting increases the likelihood that the child will understand and respond appropriately. Use this technique when talking with the child, giving the child directions, correcting the child's behavior, or when teaching the child in formal situations. Its use increases the communication partner's confidence in handling the child's misbehavior and helps eliminate frustration on the part of both the child and the communication partner.

Use of the AAI technique by those interacting with the child on a daily basis increases the number of successful communication exchanges the child experiences throughout the day. The communication partner and the child are more likely to increase the amount of time they spend engaging in language-learning activities. This in turn increases the number of language-learning opportunities available to the child, which results in improvement of language-processing skills, and the child can take advantage of the language-learning opportunities that occur within his or her natural environment.

Teaching the family and other communication partners to use the AAI technique is a simple process. After determining the beginning sublevel of instruction in a Language Web, relay to the

Introduction

child's communication partner(s) the length of commands that the child is most successful with. For example, if the child is working at Sublevel 2 of *Level 1* (noun + noun), he or she is likely to only be processing short commands or other oral input that contains at most two elements. After sharing the length of input that the child is most likely to understand, model the AAI modifications that improve processing. It can be helpful to provide examples for how to use AAI techniques throughout the day. For example, the family could use the following to ask the child to get ready to go outside:

At a slowed rate of two syllables per second: John • put on • your red coat.

At a slowed rate of one syllable per second: Sue • go get • your green sweater.

Remind communication partners to use the AAI technique in all communication contexts, such as when reading books to the child, playing with the child, disciplining the child, and feeding the child. Not only can new vocabulary be learned, but comprehension of new grammatical constructions and connected language is enhanced when communication partners use the AAI technique. It is important to keep communication partners informed as the child's processing skills change so that they can alter the AAI technique as well as the length and complexity of the input they provide. A *Home Practice Letter* in Appendix C (p. 29) may be reproduced for your use. Complete the letter by indicating the AAI modifications to use, then sign and provide any additional information needed.

Progressing Through the Sublevels

Because each sublevel is either the introduction of a new concept or a combination and expansion of prior sublevels, most children will need to move through the sublevels in the current order of presentation. For example, a child who does not complete two-element commands with size and color will most likely not complete the longer, more complex commands at subsequent sublevels in the program. The majority of children need to move in order from their beginning sublevel of instruction to complete each subsequent sublevel. Expect that children will move through some sublevels more quickly than through others, and expect the repetition of some sublevels to be necessary.

The Processing Program–2nd Ed. does provide for flexibility of use in a number of ways. First, the beginning level of instruction for each child varies from child to child. All children do not need to start at *Level 1* and complete all the sublevels. Children do not need to complete sublevels if they demonstrate that they can process the concepts. Allow the child to move through the sublevels as his or her performance dictates. A child may also move slowly through the sublevels for a period of time and then increase the rate at which he or she completes subsequent sublevels.

Within a Language Web, reviewing or advancing sublevels is viable in some cases. For some children, the review of a prior sublevel may be necessary. For example, a child may process Sublevel 7 of *Level 1*, noun + singular/plural, and Sublevel 11, noun + (size + singular/plural), but have difficulty when combined into commands that contain noun + (size + singular/plural) + noun + (size +

#TPX-27701 *The Processing Program: Level 1–2nd Edition* • ©2012 Super Duper® Publications • www.superduperinc.com   21

The Processing Program

singular/plural) at Sublevel 12. If this occurs, you might review Sublevel 7, and then review Sublevel 11. Then reintroduce the longer commands at Sublevel 12. Advance children to higher sublevels if they demonstrate readiness for more complex commands and experience a rapid growth in language.

It is also acceptable to use the stimulus picture plates to present your own sets of commands to the child. Additionally, you might alter the language of the commands if necessary for a particular child.

Reinforcement

Many children enjoy practice activities and will complete the picture-identification tasks in *The Processing Program–2nd. Ed.* with just verbal reinforcement and encouragement. Other children might need a bit more coaxing. One incentive could be that as the children respond to commands, they earn a part to a toy that they can build at a later time. After earning all possible pieces, they can then construct the toy or take the pieces home and build the toy with a family member.

Another incentive that is particularly reinforcing to children is earning money or tokens in order to purchase items or privileges. A "treasure box" that contains a variety of toys and other items popular with children is particularly enticing. You can give a penny or token for each task completed in the program, and the child can then choose items from the box to take home after earning the agreed upon amount. Other children enjoy earning tokens to exchange for special "treats" or privileges at home (e.g., earning a breakfast alone with Mom/Dad or an ice-cream treat).

Still other children enjoy graphing their responses and monitoring their progress through the program. You can make a simple graph with the number of sessions on one axis and the child's percentage of correct responses on the other. This is also great information to have children share with their families.

Monitoring Progress

It is critical to monitor the child's responses to the commands in *The Processing Program–2nd. Ed.*. A plus-or-minus (+/-) scoring system for monitoring progress works well. Keeping a written record of the child's responses is important for several reasons:

1. The collection of data helps monitor and document progress.

2. Analysis of responses helps determine when to move the child to another sublevel or when to begin the next level within the program.

3. Analysis of responses helps determine when the parameters of the AAI need modification.

4. Record keeping ensures continuity from session to session.

Introduction

There is a blank, reproducible *Progress Sheet* in Appendix D (p. 30) for your use. The *Progress Sheet* is two pages in length. Make one copy of the first page and then as many copies of the second page as you need for each child. To use the form, complete the identifying information at the top of the first page for each child. To record data, note the date of the child's session in the *Date* column on the form. In the *Sublevel and Concepts* column, record the sublevel at which the child is working and the sublevel concepts emphasized. Abbreviations, such as the following, are useful:

n = noun   s/p = singular/plural   s = size   c = color   p = preposition   q = quantity

lf = line form   t = temporal   cond. = conditional   pos. = position

Next, check the appropriate column to indicate the AAI technique in use at that sublevel. For example, if there is an alteration in speech rate, place an X in the *Rate* column, if there is alteration of speech rate and pausing, place an X in the *Rate* column and *Pausing* column. Finally, if there is alteration of speech rate, pausing, and prosody, place an X in each of the three columns for *Rate*, *Pausing*, and *Prosody*.

After the child responds to each command within a sublevel, record the response using a plus or minus (+/-). Compute a percentage of correct responses after each set of 10 commands. This may or may not correspond to the number of commands provided at a particular sublevel in the program; therefore, there may need to be a repetition of commands in order to derive 10 items. When the child's percentage of correct responses increases to 100% on 10 items at a particular sublevel, and you begin to fade the use of the AAI, indicate that on the form also.

Figure 1 on page 24 is an example of a partially completed *Progress Sheet*. In **Figure 1**, note that for the first three sets of 10 commands, at *Level 2* , Sublevel 6 (color + noun), the AAI modifications of slowing rate of speech, altering pausing, and altering prosody were necessary. By the third set of 10 commands, A.C.'s performance had reached 100% and fading of the AAI technique began at that sublevel. On the next set, the commands were presented with only slowed speech and altered pausing. By the fifth set of 10, only slowed speech was needed; by the sixth set, the commands were presented at a normal speaking rate with normal pausing and prosody. Note that by session 6, A.C. completed 100% of the items given, the AAI technique was no longer needed, and he was ready to move to the next sublevel (i.e., *Level 2, Sublevel 7, Plate 1*, size + color + noun). Remember that the number of items the child needs in order to move to the next sublevel does not correspond to the number of items at a sublevel. It is sometimes necessary to repeat commands at a sublevel until the child reaches the criterion level.

For more information regarding the progress children demonstrate when participating in *The Processing Program–2nd. Ed.*, see the discussion presented in *Outcomes* in Appendix E (pp. 32–33). The discussion presents overall anecdotal observations and standardized test data from a case study.

#TPX-27701 *The Processing Program: Level 1–2nd Edition* • ©2012 Super Duper® Publications • www.superduperinc.com

The Processing Program

Figure 1

Example Progress Sheet

Progress Sheet

Child's Name: _A.C._　　　School: _Sunset Elementary_

Birth Date: _12/1/93_　　　Grade: _2nd_

Age: _7 years, 5 months_　　　Level:　1　②　3

Date	Sublevel - Plate and Concepts	AAI Technique			Child's Responses	Percent Correct
		Rate	Pausing	Prosody		
1/7	6-1: c + n	X	X	X	+ - - + + + + + + +	80%
1/7	6-2: c + n	X	X	X	+ + + + + - + + + +	90%
1/14	6-3: c + n	X	X	X	+ + + + + + + + + +	100%
1/14	6-4: c + n	X	X		+ + + + + + + + + +	100%
1/14	6-5: c + n	X			+ + + + + + + + + +	100%
1/21	6-6: c + n				+ + + + + + + + + +	100%
1/21	7-1: s + c + n	X	X	X	- + + + + - + + + +	80%

n = noun　s/p = singular/plural　s = size　c = color　p = preposition　q = quantity
lf = line form　t = temporal　cond. = conditional　pos. = position

24　#TPX-27701 *The Processing Program: Level 1–2nd Edition* • ©2012 Super Duper® Publications • www.superduperinc.com

Appendices

Appendix A

Summary of AAI Technique Use

1. Begin at a sublevel in which the child completes at least 80% of the commands correctly at a normal speaking rate.

2. Increase correct responses to 100% at this sublevel while using the AAI technique:

   a. Slow your speaking rate.

   b. If necessary, add pauses to the slowed speaking rate.

   c. If necessary, increase or decrease prosody while pausing and using a slowed speaking rate.

3. Repeat commands at the sublevel while fading use of the AAI technique but maintaining 100% accuracy.

4. Fade use of AAI technique by:

   a. Returning prosody to normal (if applicable).

   b. Eliminating pauses (if applicable).

   c. Increasing speaking rate to normal.

5. Advance the child to the next sublevel, but return to using the AAI technique by first slowing, then adding pauses, then altering prosody to maintain 80% or better accuracy at the new sublevel.

6. Gradually decrease use of the AAI technique as the child's processing performance improves.

#TPX-27701 *The Processing Program: Level 1–2nd Edition* • ©2012 Super Duper® Publications • www.superduperinc.com

Appendix B

Determining your Natural Speaking Rate

Here is a way to determine your natural speaking rate. Time yourself while saying the Pledge of Allegiance twice and adding "I'm done" to the end. This is exactly 100 syllables. Divide 100 by your time to get your syllable-per-second rate. For example, if you say the Pledge two times, plus "I'm done," in 25 seconds, your syllable per second rate of speech would be 4.0.

Script with 100 syllables:

I pledge allegiance to the flag

Of the United States of America,

And to the republic for which it stands,

One nation, under God, indivisible,

With liberty and justice for all.

I pledge allegiance to the flag

Of the United States of America,

And to the republic for which it stands,

One nation, under God, indivisible,

With liberty and justice for all.

I'm done.

Appendix C

Home Practice Letter

Dear Family,   Date: _____

The following simple technique may help your child understand and use language easier and more accurately. It is called the Altered Auditory Input (AAI) technique. The AAI technique involves modifying:

- The speed with which you talk.
- The pauses you use when you talk.
- The melody of your speech.

Your child might better understand what you say if you shorten your sentences and speak using simpler language. In addition, it may help if you make one or more of the following changes in your speech when you are talking:

☐ Slow your rate of talking. A rate like that of Mr. Rogers is usually slow enough for most children. You may need to speak even slower though. Experiment with different slowed speaking rates and pay attention to what works best for your child.

☐ Slow your rate of speaking and add more pauses than you normally would. For example, if you want your child to clean up his/her toys, you might add the following pauses (note that you are slowing your speaking and adding pauses at the dots [•]):

Pick up • your red car.

Pick up • your • red car.

Pick • up • your • red • car.

☐ Slow your rate of speaking, add more pauses, and increase or decrease the "melody" of your speech. You do this by either talking in a monotone, a more robot-like voice, or a singsong voice, like when you are trying to hold the attention of a child while reading a storybook.

There may be changes to the AAI technique as your child's language skills improve. If you have any questions, call me _____.

Sincerely,

_____

#TPX-27701 *The Processing Program: Level 1–2nd Edition* • ©2012 Super Duper® Publications • www.superduperinc.com   29

Appendix D

Progress Sheet

Child's Name: _____   School: _____

Birth Date: _____   Grade: _____

Age: _____   Level: 1   2   3

Date	Sublevel – Plate and Concepts	AAI Technique			Child's Responses	Percent Correct
		Rate	Pausing	Prosody		

n = noun   s/p = singular/plural   s = size   c = color   p = preposition   q = quantity

lf = line form   t = temporal   cond. = conditional   pos. = position

Appendix D

Progress Sheet

Date	Sublevel – Plate and Concepts	AAI Technique			Child's Responses	Percent Correct
		Rate	Pausing	Prosody		

#TPX-27701 *The Processing Program: Level 1–2nd Edition* • ©2012 Super Duper® Publications • www.superduperinc.com

Appendix E

Outcomes

At present, there is no formal clinical research using standard methods of investigation on the efficacy of *The Processing Program*. However, pre- and posttest scores and written data have been recorded for children participating in the program. Some of these data are standardized test scores and some are anecdotal observations.

The first edition of *The Processing Program* was used with children in public school, outpatient rehabilitation, and private practice settings. The children presented with a wide range of diagnoses, including severe multiple disabilities and children with less severe difficulties. *The Processing Program* was always used in combination with other intervention activities. The typical use of the program was during the first 15–20 minutes of a session with use of the AAI technique throughout the remainder of each session. There was also teaching of the AAI technique to family members and the children's teachers whenever possible. Some put the technique to use; others did not.

Children typically received intervention at least once per week. The most effective combination of use seemed to be when *The Processing Program* was used with the child two or more times per week, and the child's communication partners used the AAI technique daily. In this case, improvement in language processing and language comprehension was usually seen within the first week of intervention. If *The Processing Program* was used only during formal intervention sessions, and the communication partners did not use the AAI technique, positive changes typically occurred within the first two months of intervention (i.e., 8–12 hours of total contact time with the child).

Changes in a number of language and associated behaviors were nearly always observed with use of *The Processing Program*. The following types of changes were often observed.

Receptive Language
- An increase in appropriate responses to questions
- An increase in understanding commands containing age-appropriate concepts
- A decrease in response delay
- An increase in receptive vocabulary
- An increase in length and complexity of commands processed

Expressive Language
- An increase in intelligibility of single words
- An increase in the number of syllables in multisyllabic words
- An increase in the child's marking of word boundaries within multiword utterances
- An increase in the mean length of utterances (MLUs)

Associated Behaviors
- A decrease in echolalia (when present)
- An increase in appropriate eye contact

Appendix E

Not all children improved in all areas, but all children seemed to improve in at least one area. The majority of children improved in the areas of communication that required remediation. The following case study illustrates changes observed while using Level 1 of *The Processing Program.*

Case Study

When K.W. was first referred at age 4 years, 1 month, he had a history of speech and language delays, particularly expressive language delays and auditory processing problems; attention problems; and fine and gross motor difficulties. Overall cognitive skills appeared to be within normal limits. He was seen once weekly for a one-hour session. Additional intervention activities were used when time permitted. He was dismissed from intervention when he was 5 years, 5 months. He made the following gains during the course of intervention:

Preschool Language Scale–3 (Zimmerman, Steiner, & Pond, 1992)

Auditory Comprehension

Chronological Age	Language Equivalency
4 years, 1 month	4 years, 0 months
4 years, 8 months	4 years, 11 months
5 years, 0 months	5 years, 4 months
5 years, 5 months	6 years, 9 months

Expressive Communication

Chronological Age	Language Equivalency
4 years, 1 month	3 years, 0 months
4 years, 8 months	3 years, 3 months
5 years, 0 months	4 years, 2 months
5 years, 5 months	5 years, 6 months

Expressive One-Word Picture Vocabulary Test (Gardner, 1981)

Chronological Age	Mental Age
5 years, 0 months	6 years, 7 months

The Token Test for Children (DiSimoni, 1978)

Chronological Age	Number Correct (of 61)	Standard Score	Standard Deviation (SD) from the Mean
4 years, 1 month	17	492	1 SD below mean
4 years, 7 months	28	496	Within 1 SD of the mean
5 years, 0 months	46	502	1 SD above the mean

When dismissed, K.W.'s receptive and expressive language skills tested in the normal range. He continued to have a mild-moderate articulation disorder, but his overall speech intelligibility was good.

#TPX-27701 *The Processing Program: Level 1–2nd Edition* • ©2012 Super Duper® Publications • www.superduperinc.com

References

Alloway, T. P. (2009). Working memory, but not IQ, predicts subsequent learning in children with learning difficulties. *European Journal of Psychological Assessment, 25*, 92–98.

Brady, S. A. (1997). Ability to encode phonological representations: An underlying difficulty of poor readers. In B.A. Blachman (Ed.), *Foundations of reading acquisition and dyslexia: Implications for early intervention* (pp. 21–47). Mahwah, NJ: Erlbaum.

Boudreau, D., & Constanza-Smith, A. (2011). Assessment and treatment of working memory deficits in school-age children: The role of the speech-language pathologist. *Language, Speech, and Hearing Services in Schools, 42*, 152–166.

Catts, H. (1997). Early identification of language-based reading disabilities. *Language, Speech, and Hearing Services in Schools, 28*, 86–87.

Cognitive Concepts. (1997). *Earobics®* [Computer software]. Evanston, IL: Author.

Deevy, P., & Leonard, L. (2004). The comprehension of Wh questions in children with specific language impairment. *Journal of Speech, Language, and Hearing Research, 47*, 802–815.

Disimoni, E. (1978). *The Token Test for Children*. Allen, TX: DLM Teaching Resources.

Dun, L., & Dunn, L. (1981). *Peabody Picture Vocabulary Test-Revised*. Circle Pines, MN: American Guidance Service.

Ellis Weismer, S. (1996). Capacity limitations in working memory: The impact on lexical and morphological learning by children with language impairment. *Topics in Language Disorders, 17*(1), 33–44.

Ellis Weismer, S. (1997). Stress in language processing. *Topics in Language Disorders, 17*(4), 41–52 .

Ellis Weismer, S., & Hesketh, L. (1996). Lexical learning by children with specific language impairment: Effects of linguistic input presented at varying speaking rates. *Journal of Speech, Language, and Hearing Research, 39*, 177–190.

Ellis Weismer, S., & Hesketh, L. (1998). The impact of emphatic stress on novel word learning by children with speech-language impairment. *Journal of Speech, Language, and Hearing Research, 41*, 1444–1457.

Gardner, M. F. (1981). *Expressive One-Word Picture Vocabulary Test*. Novato, CA: Academic Therapy.

Gillam, R.B., Cowan, N., & Marler, J.A. (1998). Information processing by school-age children with specific language impairment: Evidence from a modality effect paradigm. *Journal of Speech, Language, and Hearing Research, 41*, 913–926.

Gillam, R., Loeb, D., Hoffman, L., Bohman, T., Champlin, C., & Thibodeau, L. (2008). The efficacy of Fast ForWord language intervention in school-age children with language impairment: A randomized controlled trial. *Journal of Speech, Language, and Hearing Research, 51*, 97–199.

Just, M., & Carpenter, P. (1992). A capacity theory of comprehension: Individual differences in working memory. *Psychological Review, 99*, 122–149.

Kamhi, A. J., Catts, H. W., & Davis, M. K. (1984). Management of sentence production demands. *Journal of Speech, Language, and Hearing Research, 27,* 329–338.

McKinnis, S., & Thompson, M. (1999). Altered auditory input and language webs to improve language processing. *Language, Speech, and Hearing Services in Schools, 30,* 302–310.

Merzenich, M. M., & Jenkins, W. M. (1995). Cortical plasticity and learning: Some basic principles. In B. Jules and L. Kovacs (Eds.), *Maturational windows and adult cortical plasticity* (Vol. XXII, pp. 247–272). San Francisco, CA: Addison-Wesley.

Merzenich, M. M., Jenkins, W. M., Johnston, P., Schreiner, C., Miller, S. L., & Tallal, P. (1996). Temporal processing deficits of language-learning impaired children ameliorated by training. *Science, 271,* 77–80.

Merzenich, M. M., Tallal, P., Peterson, B., Miller, S., & Jenkins, W. M. (1999). Some neurological principles relevant to the origins of — and the cortical plasticity-based remediation of — developmental language impairments. In Grafman and Y. Christen (Eds.), *Neuronal plasticity: Building a bridge from the laboratory to the clinic* (pp. 169–187). New York: Springer-Verlag.

Montgomery, J. (2002). Understanding the language difficulties of children with specific language impairments: Does verbal working memory matter? *American Journal of Speech-Language Pathology, 11,* 77–91.

Montgomery, J. & Evans, J. (2009). Complex sentence comprehension and working memory in children with specific language impairment. *Journal of Speech, Language, and Hearing Research, 52,* 269–288.

Montgomery, J., Magimairaj, B., & Finney, M. (2010). Working memory and specific language impairment: An update on the relation and perspectives on assessment and treatment. *American Journal of Speech-Language Pathology, 19,* 78–94.

Nicolosi, L., Harryman, E., & Kresheck, J. (1989). *Terminology of communication disorders: Speech-language-hearing* (3rd ed.). Baltimore: Williams and Wilkins.

Porch, B. E. (1979). *Porch index of communicative ability in children.* Chicago: Riverside Publishing.

Rice, M. L., Buhr, J. C., & Nemeth, M. (1990). Fast mapping word-learning abilities of language delayed preschoolers. *Journal of Speech, Language, and Hearing Disorders, 55,* 33–90.

Robin, D., Tomblin, B., Kearney, A., & Hug, L. (1989). Auditory temporal pattern learning in children with speech and language impairments. *Brain and Language, 36,* 604–613.

Scientific Learning. (1998). *Fast ForWord®* [Computer software]. Berkeley, CA: Author.

Shankweiler, D., Crain, S., Brady, S., & Macaruso, P. (1992). Identifying the causes of reading disability. In P. B. Gough, L. C. Ehri, and R. Treiman (Eds.), *Reading acquisition* (pp. 275–305). Hillsdale, NJ: Erlbaum.

Studdert-Kennedy, M., & Mody, M. (1995). Auditory temporal perception deficits in the reading-impaired: A critical review of the evidence. *Psychonomic Bulletin and Review, 2,* 508–514.

Tallal, P. (1975). Perceptual and linguistic factors in the language impairment of developmental dysphasic: An experimental investigation with the Token Test. *Cortex, 11,* 196–205.

The Processing Program

Tallal, P. (1976). Rapid auditory processing in normal and disordered language development. *Journal of Speech, Language, and Hearing Research, 19*, 561–571.

Tallal, P. (1990). Fine-grained discrimination deficits in language-learning impaired children are specific neither to the auditory modality nor to speech perception. *Journal of Speech, Language, and Hearing Research, 33*, 616–617.

Tallal, P., Miller, S. L., Bedi, G., Byma, G., Wang, X., Nagaraja, S. S., Schreiner, C. Jenkins, W. M., & Merzenich, M. M. (1996). Language comprehension in language-learning impaired children improved with acoustically modified speech. *Science, 271*, 81–84.

Tallal, P., & Newcombe, F. (1978). Impairment of auditory perception and language comprehension in dysphasia. *Brain and Language, 5*, 13–24.

Tallal, P., & Piercy, M. (1973a). Defects of non-verbal auditory perception in children with developmental aphasia. *Nature, 241*, 468–469.

Tallal, P., & Piercy, M. (1973b). Developmental aphasia: Impaired rate of non-verbal processing as a function of sensory modality. *Neuropsychological, 11*, 389–398.

Tallal, P., & Piercy, M. (1974). Developmental aphasia: Rate of auditory processing and selective impairment of consonant perception. *Neuropsychological, 12*, 83–93.

Tallal, P., & Piercy, M. (1975). Developmental aphasia: The perception of brief vowels and extended stop consonants. *Neuropsychological, 13*, 69–74.

Tallal, P., Stark, R., & Curtiss, B. (1976). Relation between speech perception and speech production impairment in children with developmental dysphagia. *Brain and Language, 3*, 305–317.

Tallal, P., Stark, R., & Mellits, E. (1985). Identification of language-impaired children on the basis of rapid perception and production skills. *Brain and Language, 25*, 314–322.

Zimmerman, I., Steiner, V., & Pond, R. (1992). *Preschool language scale—3*. San Antonio, TX: Psychological Corporation.

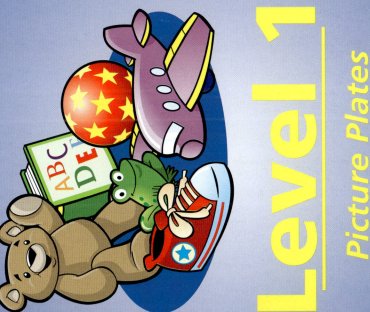

Level 1
Picture Plates

Level 1

Sublevel 1

noun

Example: *Touch the mouse.*

1. Touch the cup.
2. Touch the ball.
3. Touch the mouse.
4. Touch the cat.

Plate 1

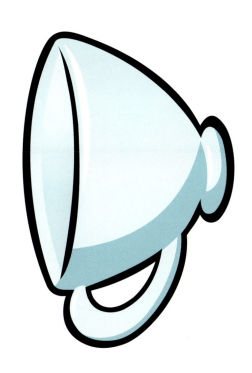
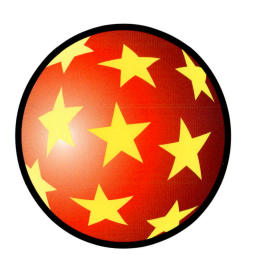

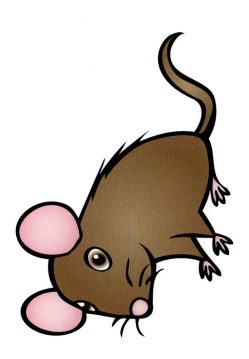
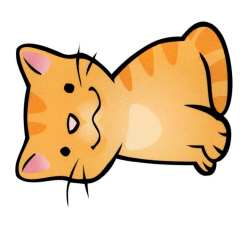

Level 1

Sublevel 1

noun

Example: *Touch the frog.*

1. Touch the dog.
2. Touch the frog.
3. Touch the duck.
4. Touch the hat.

Plate 2

©2012 Super Duper® Publications

40

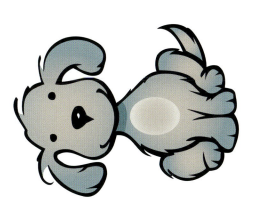
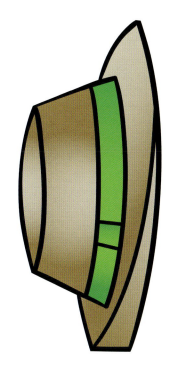
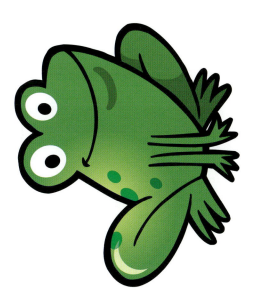
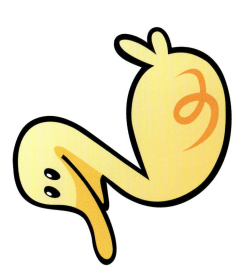
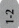

Level 1

Sublevel 1

noun

Example: *Touch the bear.*

1. Touch the bear.
2. Touch the book.
3. Touch the sock.
4. Touch the mitten.

Plate 3

©2012 Super Duper® Publications

42

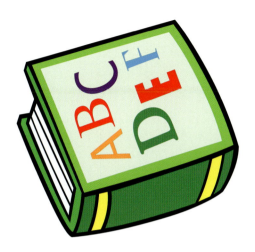
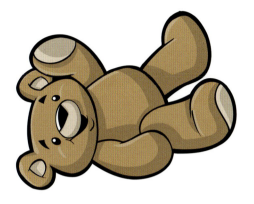
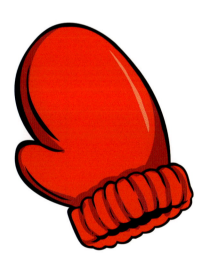
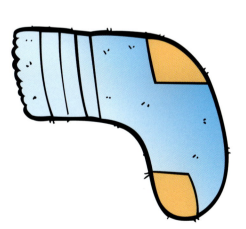

Level 1

Sublevel 1

noun

Example: *Touch the airplane.*

1. Touch the sled.
2. Touch the shoe.
3. Touch the balloon.
4. Touch the airplane.

Plate 4

©2012 Super Duper® Publications

44

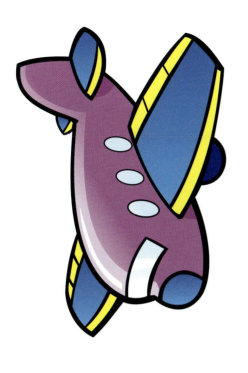
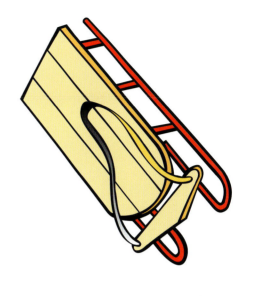
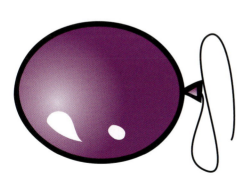
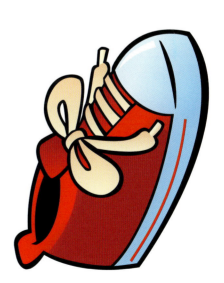
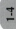

Level 1

Sublevel 1

noun

Example: *Touch the dress.*

1. Touch the bead.

2. Touch the ring.

3. Touch the dress.

4. Touch the button.

Plate 5

©2012 Super Duper® Publications

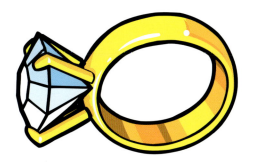
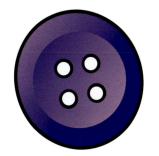
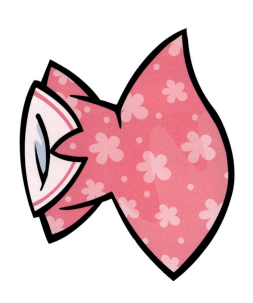
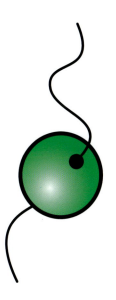

Level 1

Sublevel 2

noun + noun

Example: *Touch the cup and the balloon.*

1. Touch the cup and the balloon.
2. Touch the dog and the frog.
3. Touch the cup and the dog.
4. Touch the frog and the balloon.

Plate 1

©2012 Super Duper® Publications

48

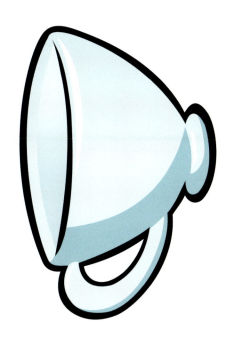
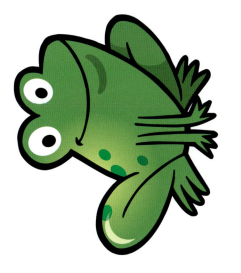
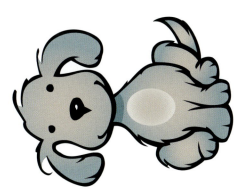
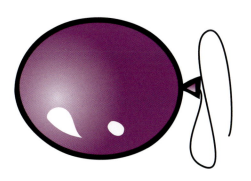
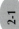

Level 1

Sublevel 2

noun + noun

Example: *Touch the cat and the hat.*

1. Touch the mouse and the ring.
2. Touch the cat and the hat.
3. Touch the cat and the mouse.
4. Touch the hat and the ring.

Plate 2

©2012 Super Duper® Publications

50

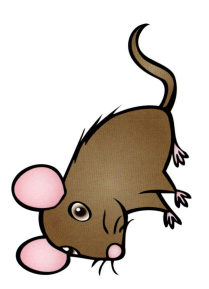
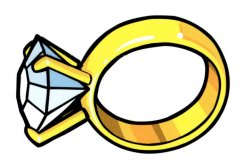
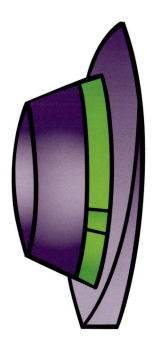
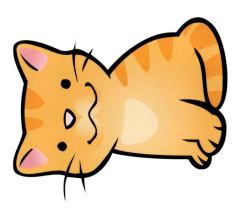
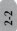

Level 1

Sublevel 2

noun + noun

Example: *Touch the ball and the airplane.*

1. Touch the duck and the bear.

2. Touch the ball and the airplane.

3. Touch the bear and the ball.

4. Touch the airplane and the duck.

©2012 Super Duper® Publications

Plate 3

52

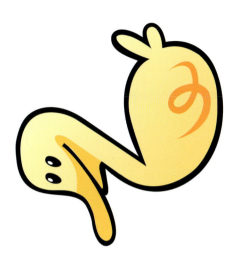
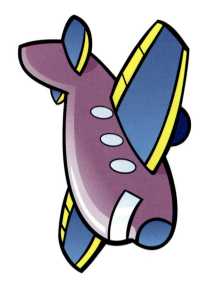
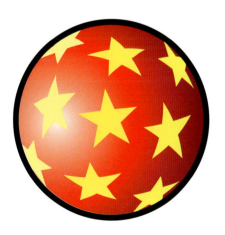
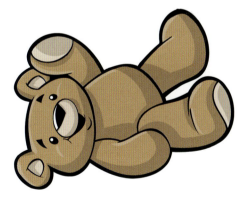

Level 1

Sublevel 2

noun + noun

Example: *Touch the bead and the mitten.*

1. Touch the sock and the bead.
2. Touch the mitten and the dress.
3. Touch the bead and the mitten.
4. Touch the dress and the sock.

Plate 4

©2012 Super Duper® Publications

54

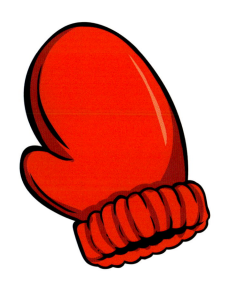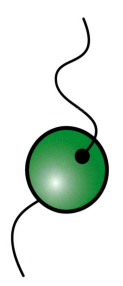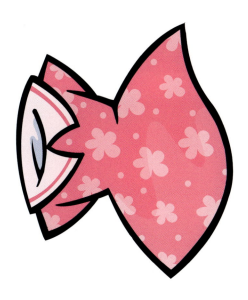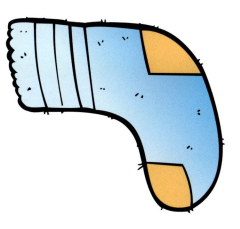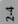

Level 1

Sublevel 2

noun + noun

Example: *Touch the book and the shoe.*

1. Touch the button and the book.
2. Touch the shoe and the ring.
3. Touch the ring and the button.
4. Touch book and the shoe.

Plate 5

©2012 Super Duper® Publications

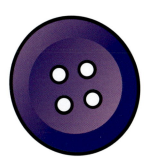
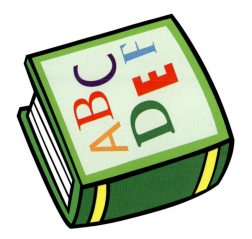
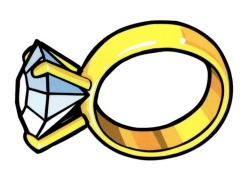
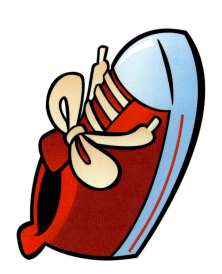

Level 1

Sublevel 2

noun + noun

Example: *Touch the bead and the frog.*

1. Touch the bead and the frog.
2. Touch the mouse and the ball.
3. Touch the frog and the mouse.
4. Touch the ball and the bead.

Plate 6

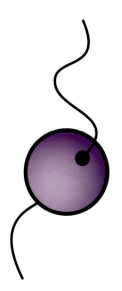
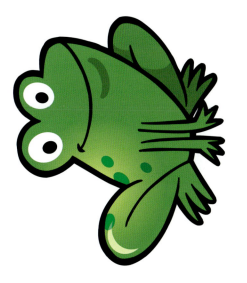
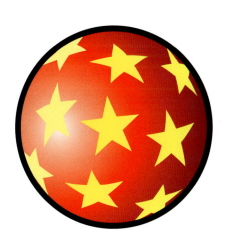
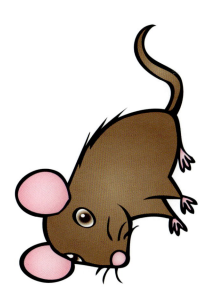

Level 1

Sublevel 2

noun + noun

Example: Touch the sled and the cat.

1. Touch the cup and the book.

2. Touch the duck and the airplane.

3. Touch the sled and the cat.

4. Touch the book and the sled.

5. Touch the airplane and the cup.

6. Touch the cat and the duck.

Plate 7

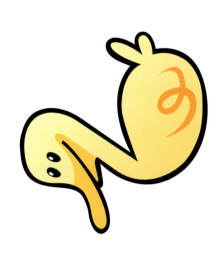
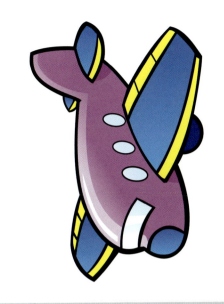
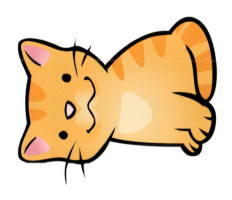
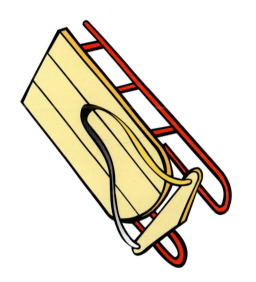
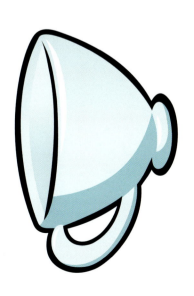
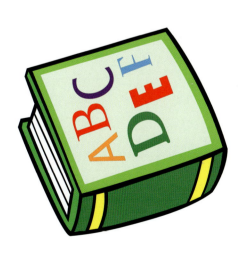

Level 1

Sublevel 2

noun + noun

Example: *Touch the ball and the hat.*

1. Touch the hat and the bead.
2. Touch the dog and the ball.
3. Touch the shoe and the sock.
4. Touch the ball and the hat.
5. Touch the sock and the dog.
6. Touch the hat and the shoe.

Plate 8

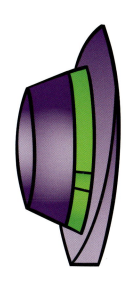
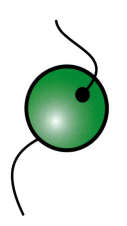
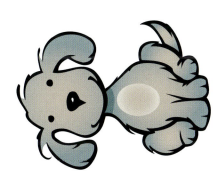
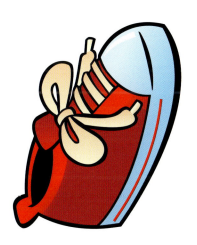
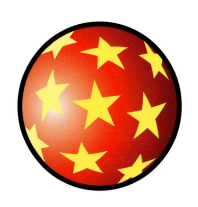
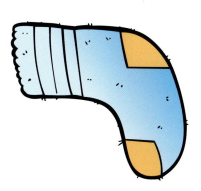

Level 1

Sublevel 2

noun + noun

Example: *Touch the mitten and the balloon.*

1. Touch the ring and the frog.
2. Touch the mouse and the mitten.
3. Touch the balloon and the bear.
4. Touch the bear and the ring.
5. Touch the mitten and the balloon.
6. Touch the frog and the mouse.

Plate 9

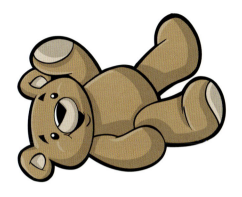
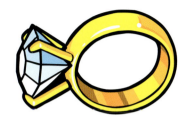
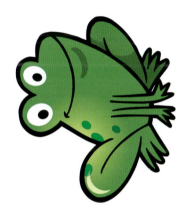
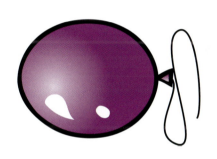
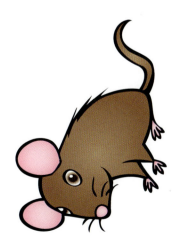
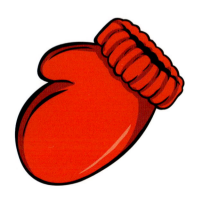

Level 1

Sublevel 2

noun + noun

Example: *Touch the cup and the hat.*

1. Touch the dress and the button.
2. Touch the frog and the cup.
3. Touch the hat and the airplane.
4. Touch the airplane and the dress.
5. Touch the button and the frog.
6. Touch the cup and the hat.

Plate 10

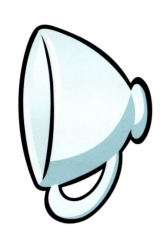
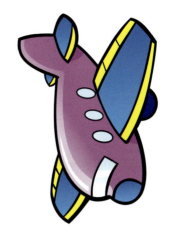
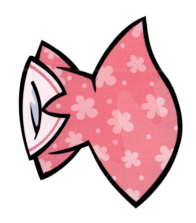
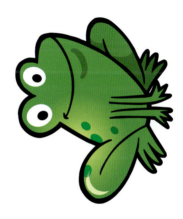

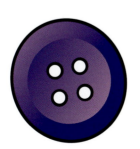
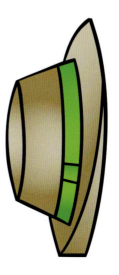

Level 1

Sublevel 3

noun + noun + noun + noun

Example: *Touch the cup with a ring, a sled, and a shoe.*

1. Touch the cup with a ball, a dog, and a mouse.

2. Touch the cup with a cat, a balloon, and an airplane.

3. Touch the cup with a frog, a bear, and a book.

4. Touch the cup with a ring, a sled, and a shoe.

Plate 1

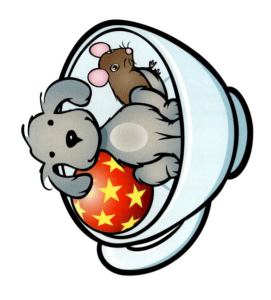
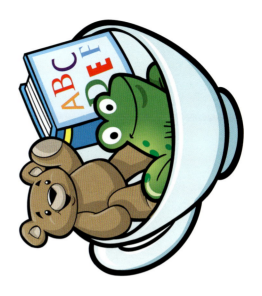
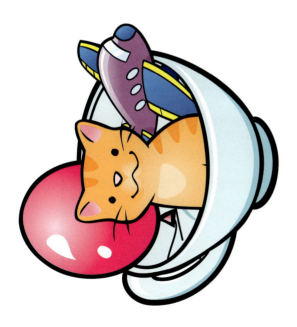
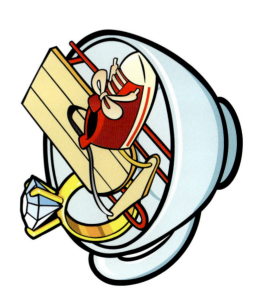
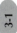

Level 1

Sublevel 3

noun + noun + noun + noun

Example: Touch the hat with a shoe, a frog, and an airplane.

1. Touch the hat with a shoe, a frog, and an airplane.
2. Touch the hat with a ball, a dress, and a mouse.
3. Touch the hat with a bead, a ring, and a cat.
4. Touch the hat with a balloon, a dog, and a button.

Plate 2

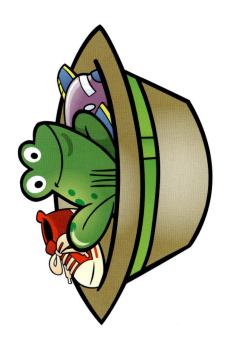
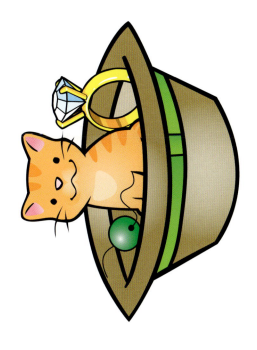
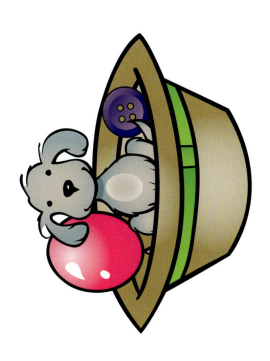
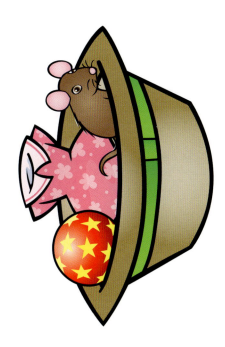
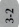

Level 1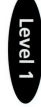

Sublevel 3

noun + noun + noun + noun

Example: *Touch the sled with a mitten, a shoe, and a button.*

1. Touch the sled with a book, a ball, and a bead.
2. Touch the sled with a ring, a sock, and a cat.
3. Touch the sled with a mitten, a shoe, and a button.
4. Touch the sled with an airplane, a frog, and a dress.

Plate 3

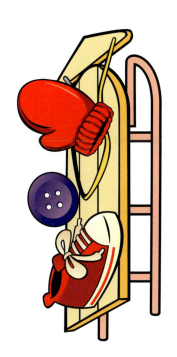
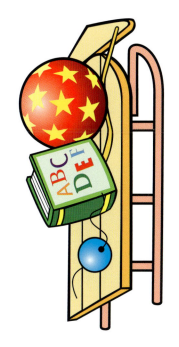
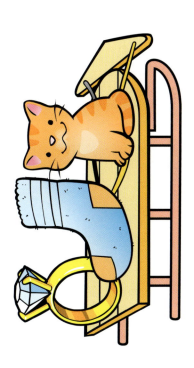
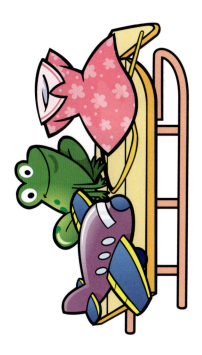
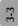

Level 1

Sublevel 3

noun + noun + noun + noun

Example: *Touch the cup with a shoe, a dress, and a bead.*

1. Touch the cup with a mitten, an airplane, and a button.

2. Touch the cup with a cat, a bear, and a dog.

3. Touch the cup with a duck, a ball, and a sock.

4. Touch the cup with a shoe, a dress, and a bead.

Plate 4

©2012 Super Duper® Publications

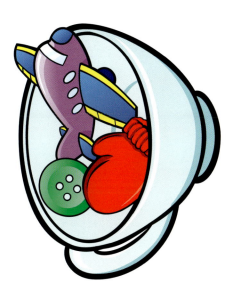
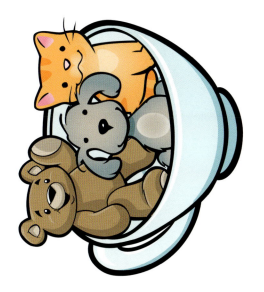
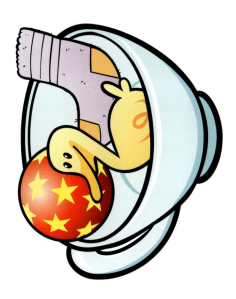
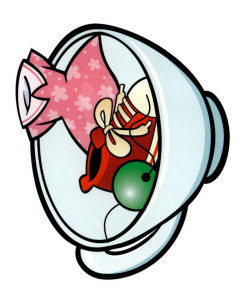

Level 1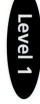

Sublevel 3

noun + noun + noun

Example: *Touch the hat with a mouse, a cat, and an airplane.*

1. Touch the hat with a mouse, a cat, and an airplane.
2. Touch the hat with a button, a ring, and a dog.
3. Touch the hat with a bear, a duck, and an airplane.
4. Touch the hat with a shoe, a dress, and a bead.

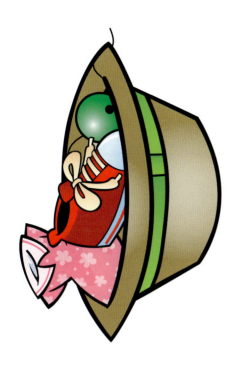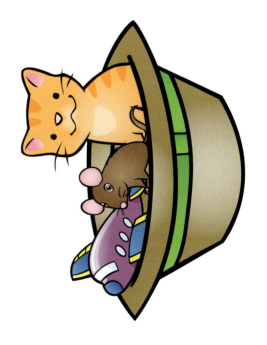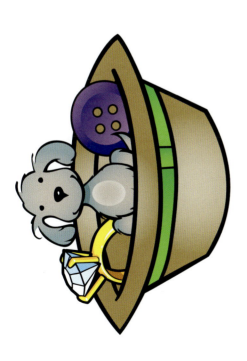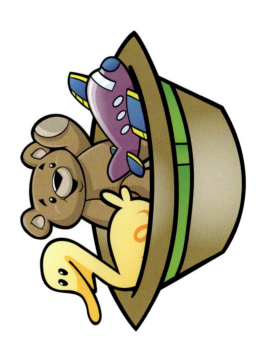

Level 1

Sublevel 3

noun + noun + noun + noun

Example: *Touch the cup with a shoe, a mitten, and a dress.*

1. Touch the hat with a bear, a mouse, and a frog.

2. Touch the cup with a shoe, a mitten, and a dress.

3. Touch the hat with a ball, a ring, and an airplane.

4. Touch the cup with a bear, a button, and a balloon.

5. Touch the hat with a sock, a cat, and a book.

6. Touch the cup with a dog, a bead, and a frog.

Plate 6

©2012 Super Duper® Publications

78

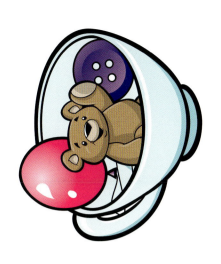
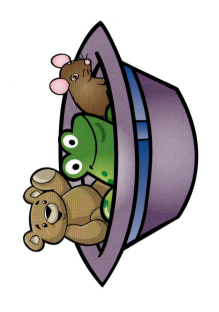
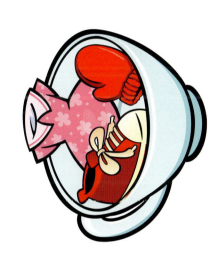
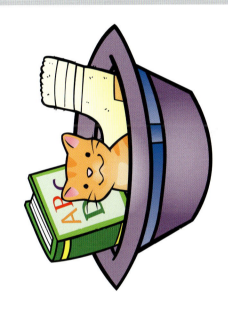
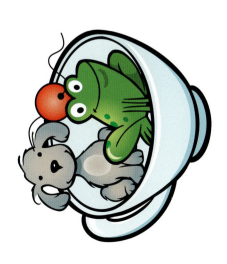
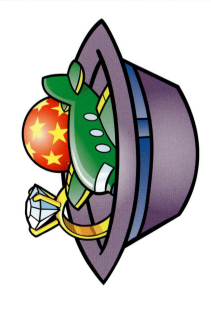

Level 1

Sublevel 3

noun + noun + noun + noun

Example: *Touch the sled with a bead, a dog, and a mouse.*

1. Touch the sled with an airplane, a shoe, and a button.

2. Touch the hat with a duck, a ball, and a cat.

3. Touch the sled with a bead, a dog, and a mouse.

4. Touch the hat with a button, a shoe, and a mouse.

5. Touch the sled with a dress, a ring, and a ball.

6. Touch the hat with a book, a mitten, and a frog.

Plate 7

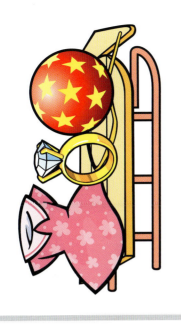
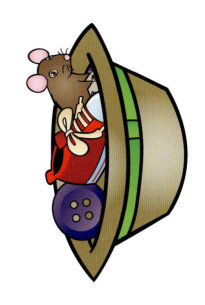
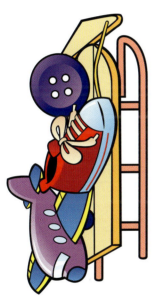
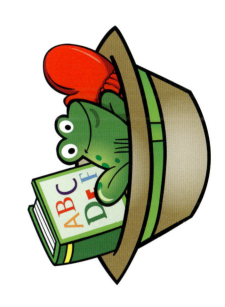
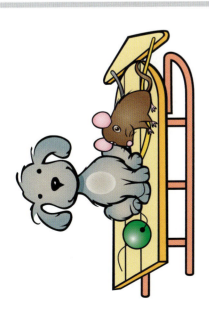
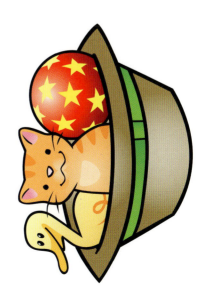

Level 1

Sublevel 3

noun + noun + noun + noun

Example: *Touch the sled with a duck, a hat, and a bead.*

1. Touch the cup with an airplane, a ball, and a shoe.

2. Touch the sled with a ball, a button, and a mouse.

3. Touch the cup with a dog, a bead, and a bear.

4. Touch the sled with a duck, a hat, and a bead.

5. Touch the cup with a dress, a ring, and a frog.

6. Touch the sled with a sock, a mitten, and a cat.

©2012 Super Duper® Publications

Plate 8

82

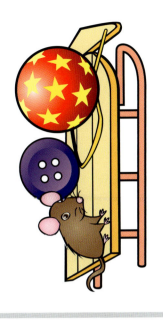
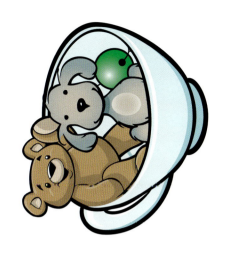
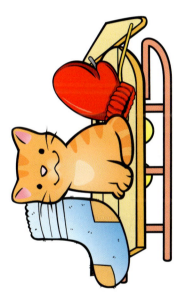
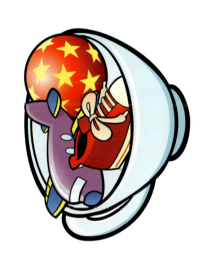
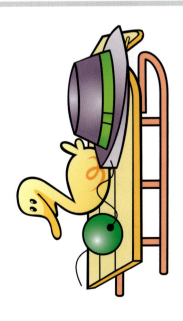
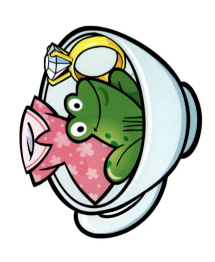

Level 1

Sublevel 3

noun + noun + noun + noun

Example: *Touch the cup with a mitten, a dress, and a ring.*

1. Touch the cup with a bear, an airplane, and a bead.

2. Touch the hat with a balloon, a book, and a ball.

3. Touch the cup with a cat, a frog, and a dog.

4. Touch the hat with a sled, a button, and a frog.

5. Touch the cup with a mitten, a dress, and a ring.

6. Touch the hat with a shoe, a duck, and a sock.

Plate 9

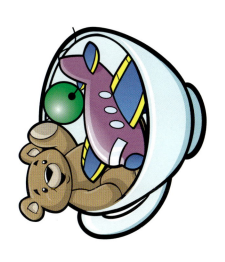
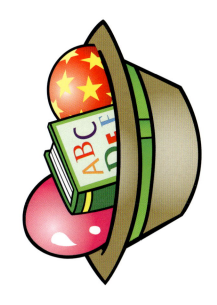
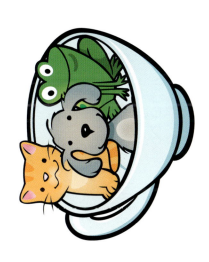
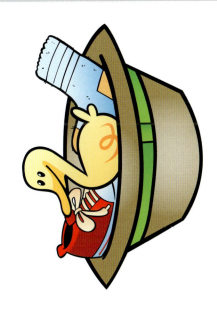
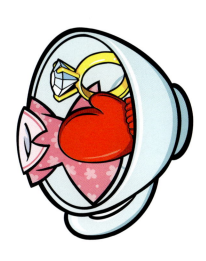
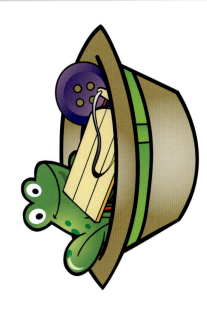

Level 1

Sublevel 3

noun + noun + noun + noun

Example: *Touch the sled with a ball, a cat, and an airplane.*

1. Touch the hat with a cup, a ring, and a dress.

2. Touch the sled with a book, a duck, and a bead.

3. Touch the hat with a sock, a mouse, and a frog.

4. Touch the sled with a bear, a button, and a shoe.

5. Touch the hat with a button, a dog, and a balloon.

6. Touch the sled with a ball, a cat, and an airplane.

Plate 10

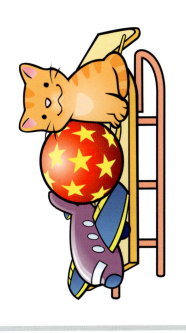
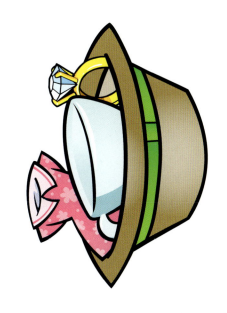
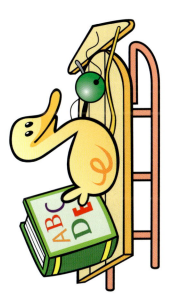
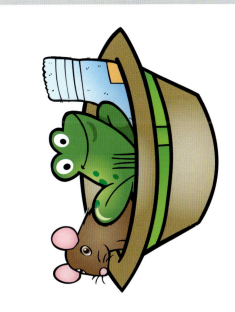
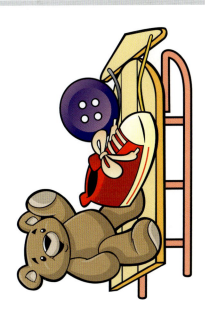
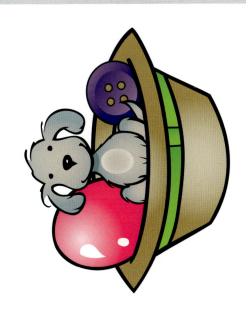
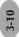

Level 1

Sublevel 4

noun + noun + noun — *first two the same*

Example: *Touch the frog, the dog, and the mouse.*

1. Touch the frog, the dog, and the hat.

2. Touch the frog, the dog, and the mouse.

3. Touch the frog, the dog, and the dress.

4. Touch the frog, the dog, and the button.

5. Touch the frog, the dog, and the duck.

6. Touch the frog, the dog, and the cat.

Plate 1

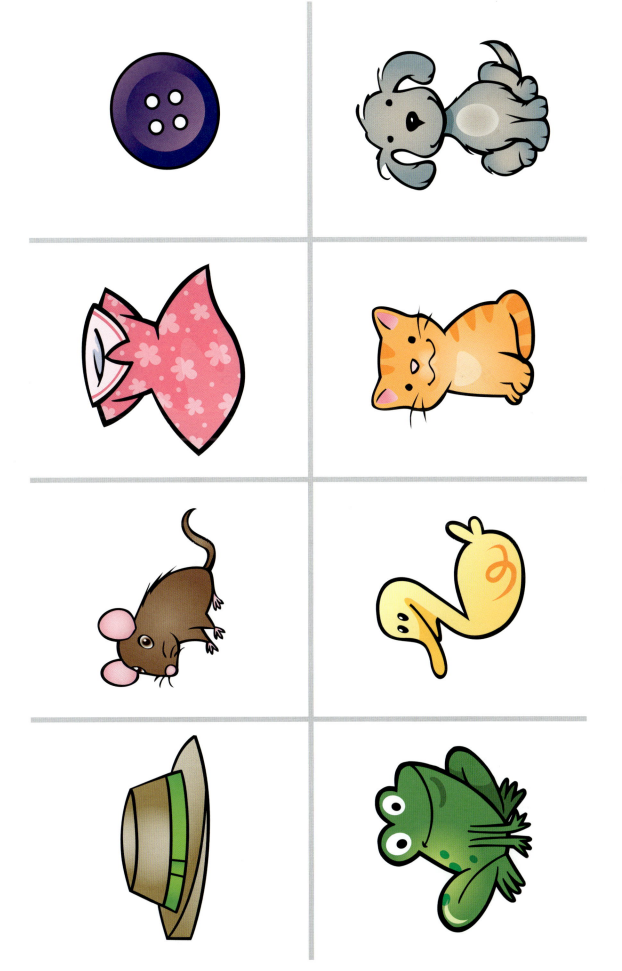

Level 1

Sublevel 4

noun + noun + noun — *first two the same*

Example: *Touch the mouse, the duck, and the dress.*

1. Touch the mouse, the duck, and the cat.

2. Touch the mouse, the duck, and the button.

3. Touch the mouse, the duck, and the hat.

4. Touch the mouse, the duck, and the dress.

5. Touch the mouse, the duck, and the frog.

6. Touch the mouse, the duck, and the dog.

Plate 2

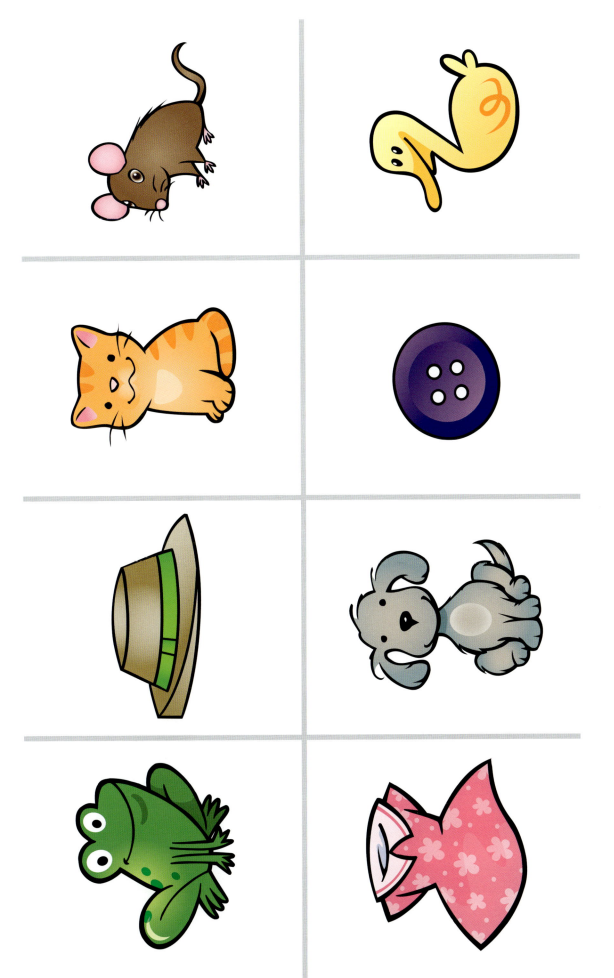

Level 1

Sublevel 4

noun + noun + noun — *first two the same*

Example: Touch the button, the cat, and the dog.

1. Touch the button, the cat, and the mouse.
2. Touch the button, the cat, and the dress.
3. Touch the button, the cat, and the duck.
4. Touch the button, the cat, and the frog.
5. Touch the button, the cat, and the dog.
6. Touch the button, the cat, and the hat.

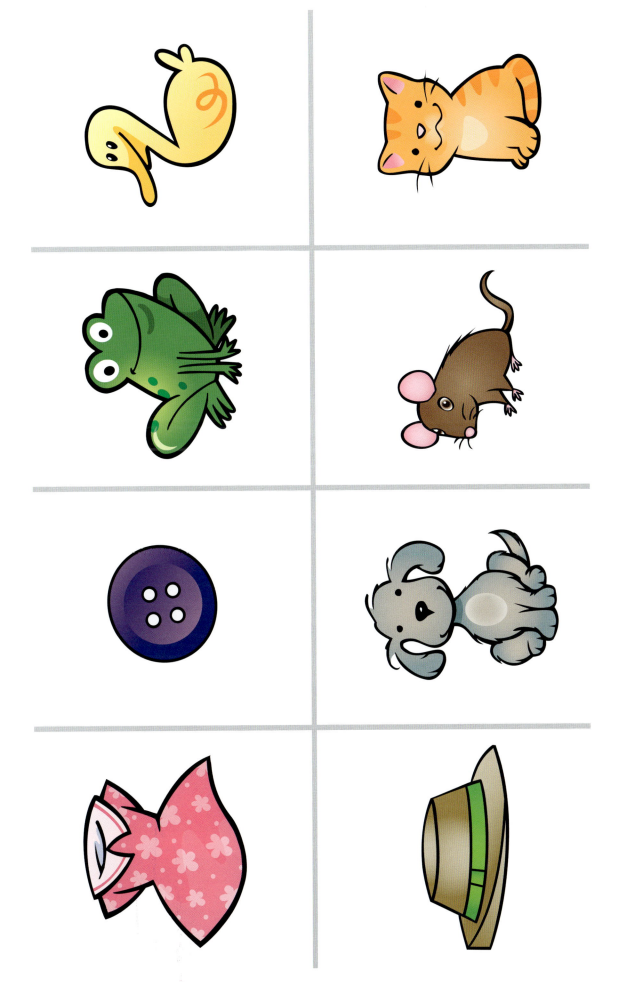

Level 1

Sublevel 4

noun + noun + noun — *first two the same*

Example: *Touch the hat, the dress, and the mouse.*

1. Touch the hat, the dress, and the dog.
2. Touch the hat, the dress, and the frog.
3. Touch the hat, the dress, and the button.
4. Touch the hat, the dress, and the cat.
5. Touch the hat, the dress, and the duck.
6. Touch the hat, the dress, and the mouse.

Plate 4

©2012 Super Duper® Publications

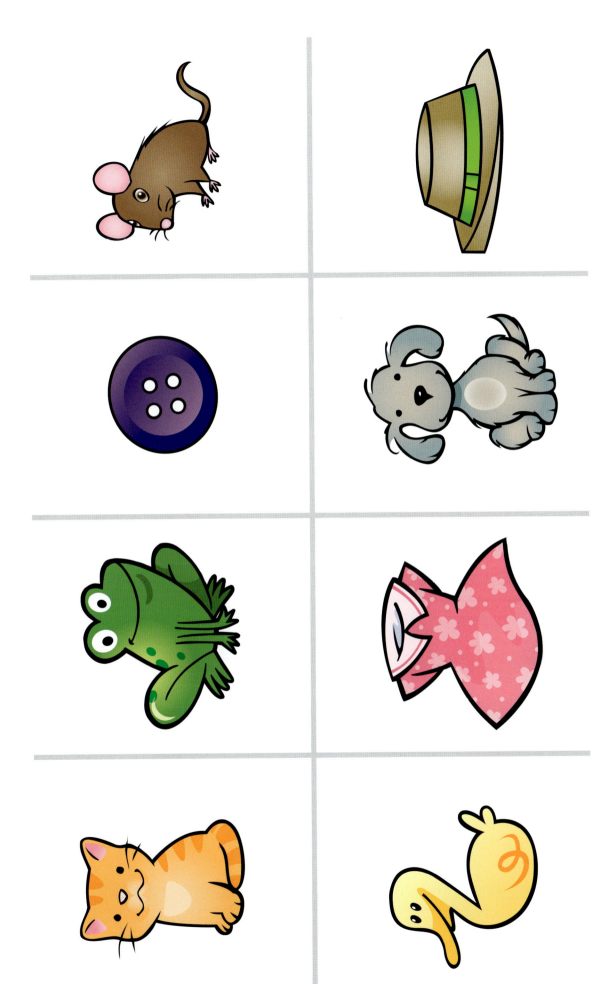

Level 1

Sublevel 5

noun + noun + noun — *first one the same*

Example: *Touch the mitten, the mouse, and the sock.*

1. Touch the mitten, the dog, and the ring.

2. Touch the mitten, the button, and the sled.

3. Touch the mitten, the mouse, and the sock.

4. Touch the mitten, the ring, and the duck.

5. Touch the mitten, the sled, and the sock.

6. Touch the mitten, the duck, and the dog.

Plate 1

©2012 Super Duper® Publications

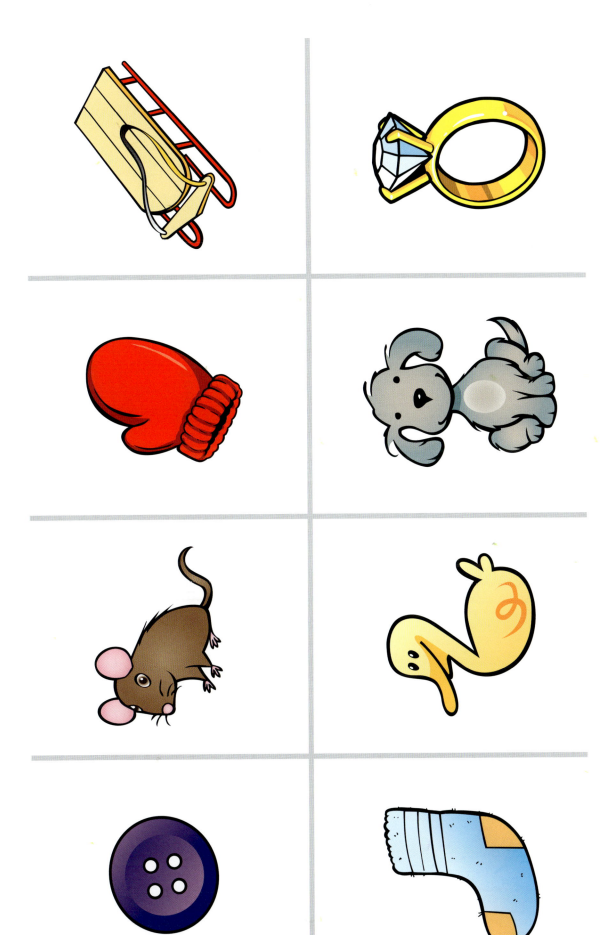

Level 1

Sublevel 5

noun + noun + noun — *first one the same*

Example: *Touch the frog, the dress, and the shoe.*

1. Touch the frog, the cup, and the bead.
2. Touch the frog, the dog, and the ball.
3. Touch the frog, the hat, and the bead.
4. Touch the frog, the dress, and the shoe.
5. Touch the frog, the shoe, and the cup.
6. Touch the frog, the ball, and the dress.

Plate 2

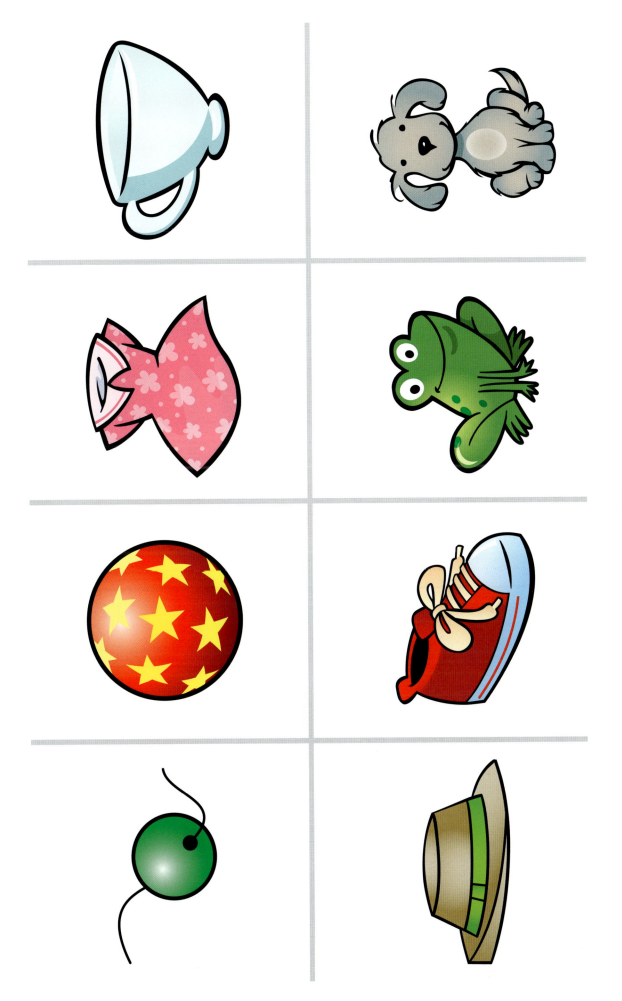

Level 1

Sublevel 5

noun + noun + noun — *first one the same*

Example: *Touch the airplane, the sock, and the cat.*

1. Touch the airplane, the ring, and the sock.
2. Touch the airplane, the bear, and the mitten.
3. Touch the airplane, the duck, and the hat.
4. Touch the airplane, the cat, and the bear.
5. Touch the airplane, the sock, and the cat.
6. Touch the airplane, the mitten, and the hat.

©2012 Super Duper® Publications

Plate 3

100

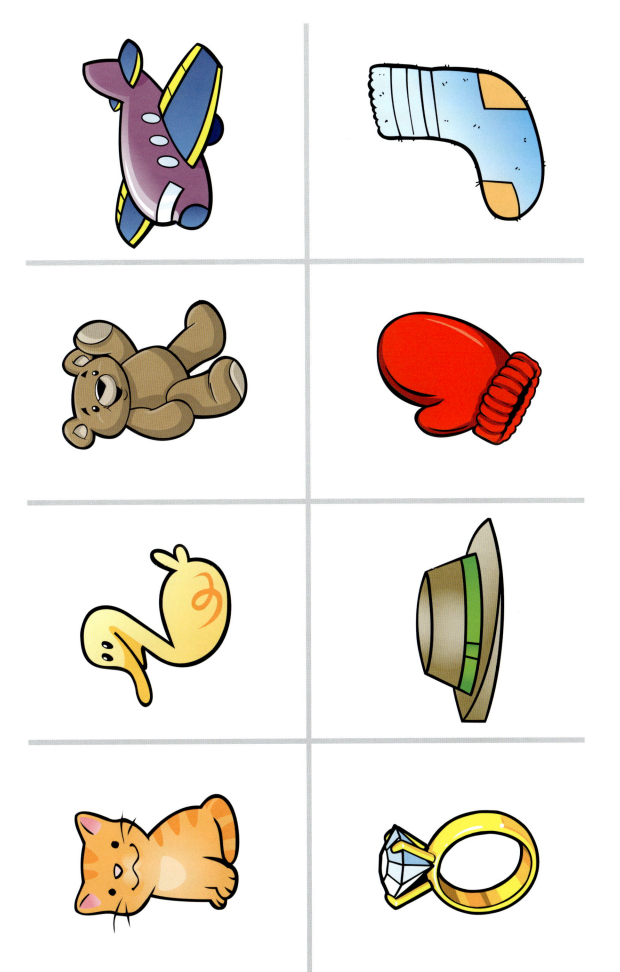

Level 1

Sublevel 5

noun + noun + noun — *first one the same*

Example: *Touch the balloon, the bead, and the shoe.*

1. Touch the balloon, the cup, and the airplane.
2. Touch the balloon, the book, and the mouse.
3. Touch the balloon, the shoe, and the ball.
4. Touch the balloon, the airplane, and the book.
5. Touch the balloon, the ball, and the cup.
6. Touch the balloon, the bead, and the shoe.

Plate 4

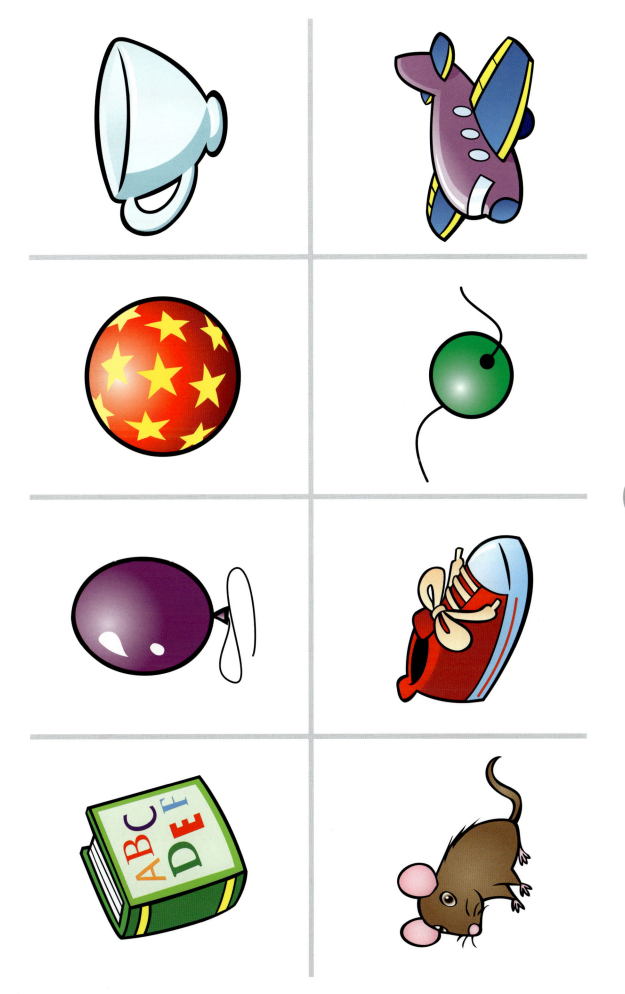

Level 1

Sublevel 6

noun + noun + noun — *all different*

Example: *Touch the dress, the sled, and the ring.*

1. Touch the duck, the frog, and the sled.

2. Touch the cat, the button, and the bead.

3. Touch the dress, the sled, and the ring.

4. Touch the bead, the frog, and the dress.

5. Touch the button, the sled, and the duck.

6. Touch the ring, the duck, and the frog.

Plate 1

©2012 Super Duper® Publications

104

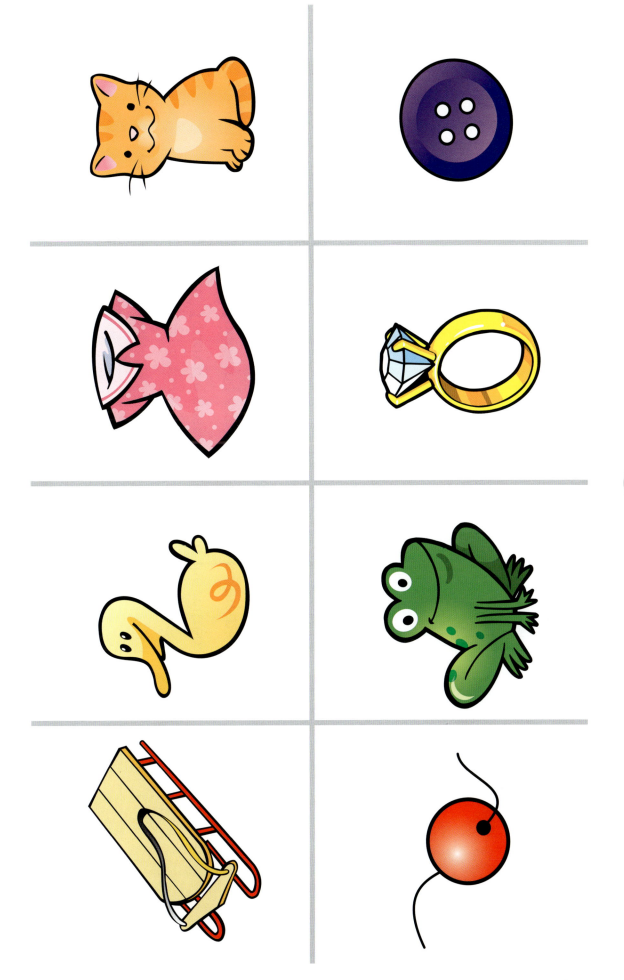

Level 1

Sublevel 6

noun + noun + noun — *all different*
Example: Touch the hat, the bear, and the balloon.

1. Touch the bear, the shoe, and the mitten.
2. Touch the airplane, the sock, and the balloon.
3. Touch the mitten, the ball, and the sock.
4. Touch the hat, the bear, and the balloon.
5. Touch the ball, the airplane, and the shoe.
6. Touch the shoe, the hat, and the bear.

Plate 2

©2012 Super Duper® Publications

106

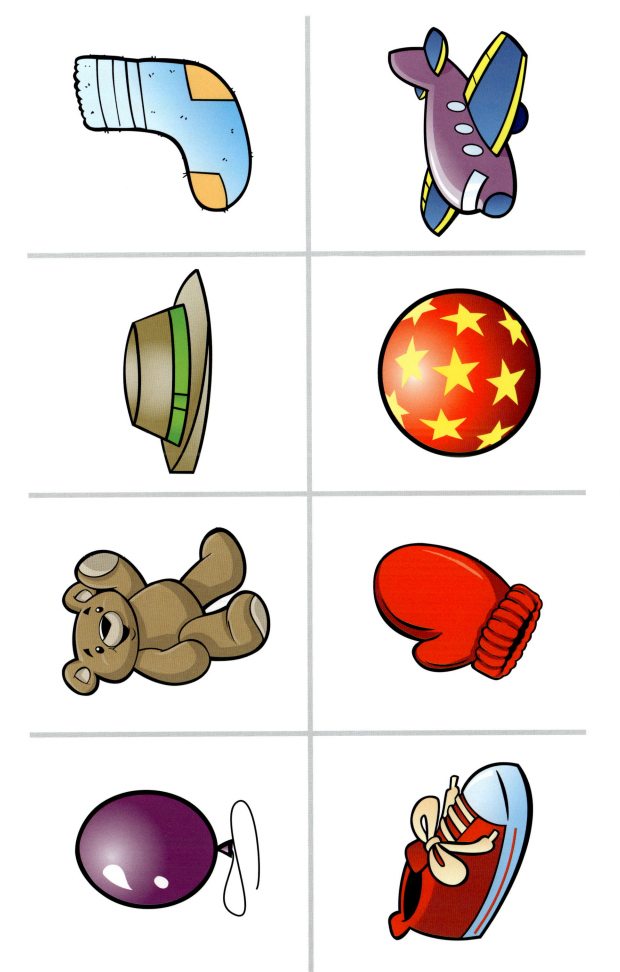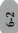

Level 1

Sublevel 6

noun + noun + noun — *all different*

Example: *Touch the dog, the book, and the mitten.*

1. Touch the sled, the dog, and the bear.
2. Touch the button, the book, and the mitten.
3. Touch the bead, the cup, and the dog.
4. Touch the sled, the button, and the cup.
5. Touch the dog, the book, and the mitten.
6. Touch the cup, the button, and the bear.

Plate 3

©2012 Super Duper® Publications

108

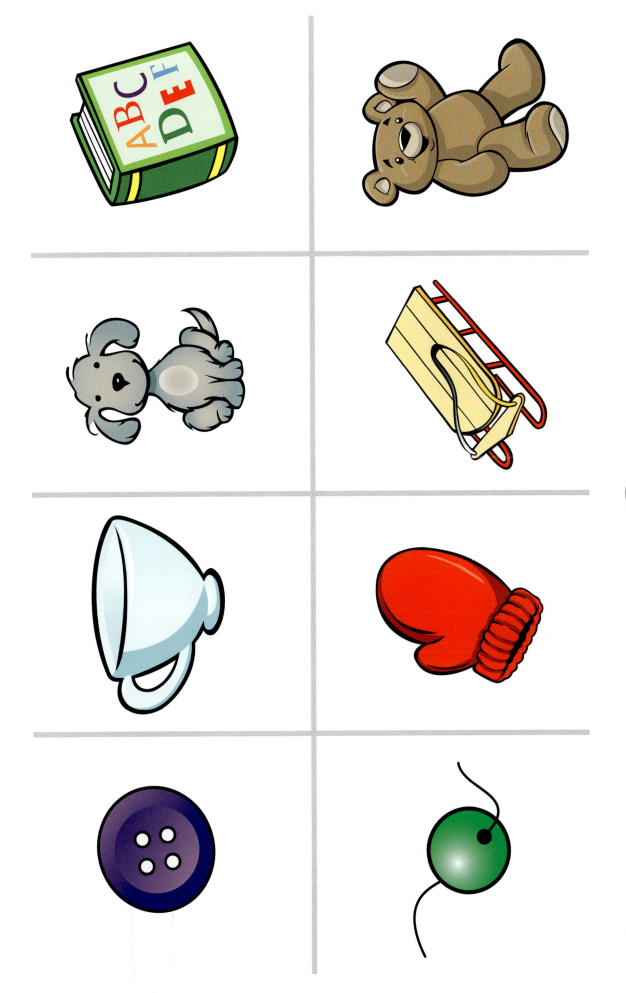

Level 1

Sublevel 6

noun + noun + noun — *all different*

Example: *Touch the duck, the hat, and the dog.*

1. Touch the mouse, the dress, and the duck.
2. Touch the hat, the airplane, and the sock.
3. Touch the dog, the ring, and the mouse.
4. Touch the sock, the dress, and the ring.
5. Touch the dress, the airplane, and the mouse.
6. Touch the duck, the hat, and the dog.

Plate 4

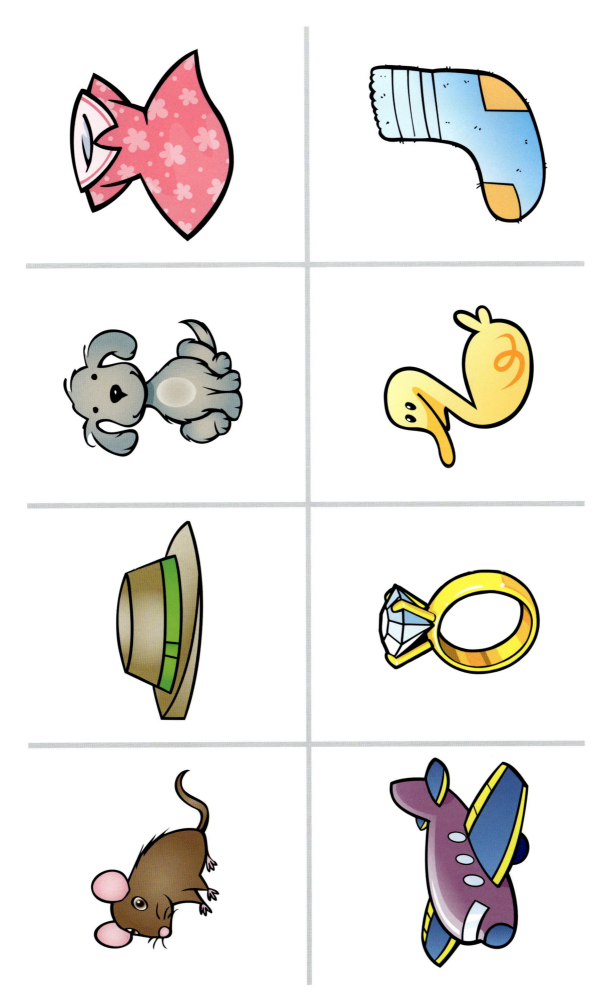

Level 1

Sublevel 7

noun + singular/plural

Example: *Touch the hat with a duck.*

1. Touch the hat with a duck.

2. Touch the cup with a cat.

3. Touch the hat with the cats.

4. Touch the cup with the ducks.

Plate 1

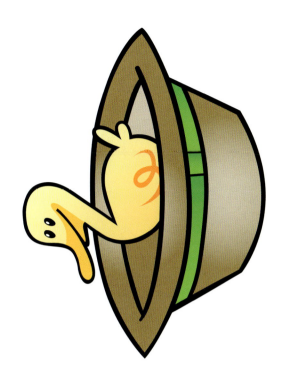
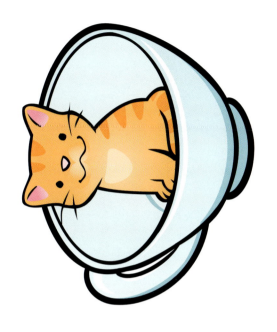
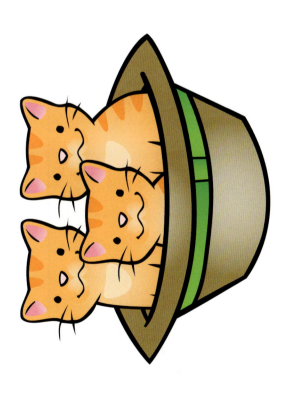
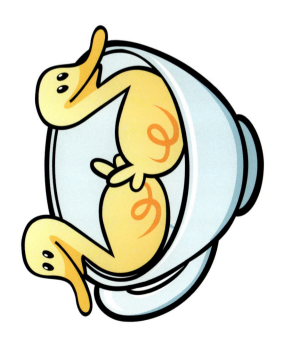

Level 1

Sublevel 7

noun + singular/plural

Example: *Touch the cup with a dress.*

1. Touch the cup with a dog.
2. Touch the cup with a dress.
3. Touch the sled with the dogs.
4. Touch the hat with the dresses.

Plate 2

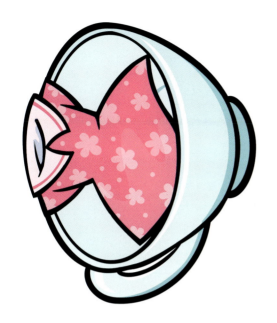
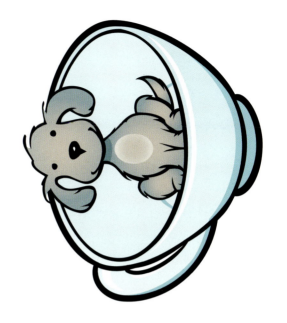
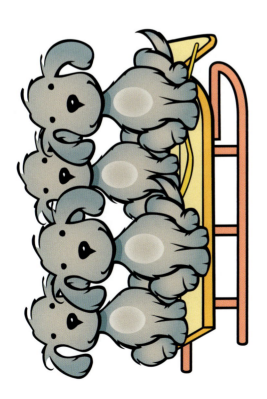
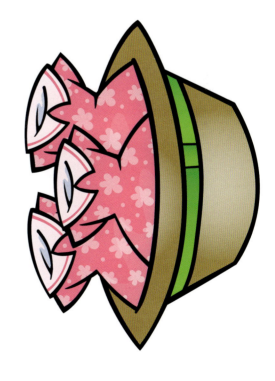

Level 1

Sublevel 7

noun + singular/plural

Example: Touch the sled with the balloons.

1. Touch the hat with a balloon.
2. Touch the hat with a shoe.
3. Touch the sled with the balloons.
4. Touch the sled with the shoes.

Plate 3

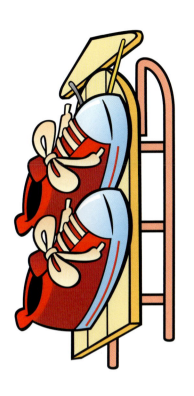
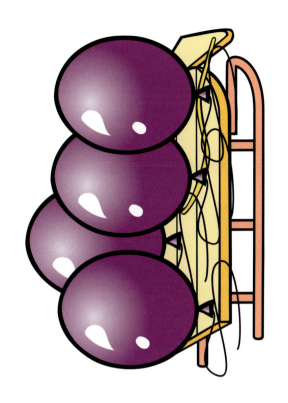
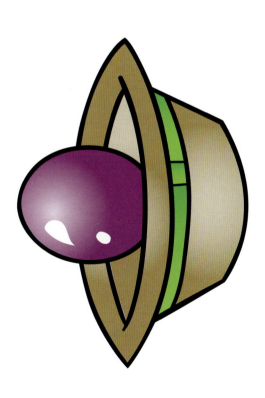
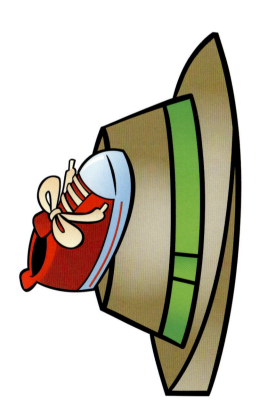

Level 1

Sublevel 7

noun + singular/plural

Example: *Touch the hat with a ball.*

1. Touch the sled with a button.
2. Touch the cup with the balls.
3. Touch the cup with the buttons.
4. Touch the hat with a ball.

Plate 4

©2012 Super Duper® Publications

118

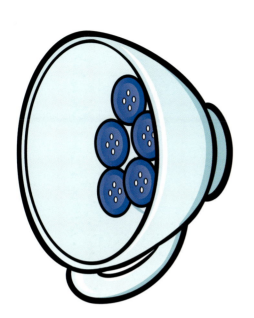
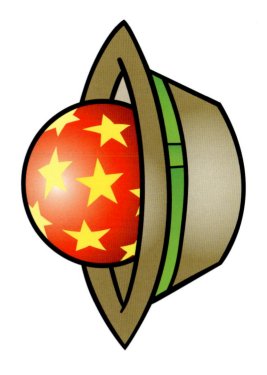
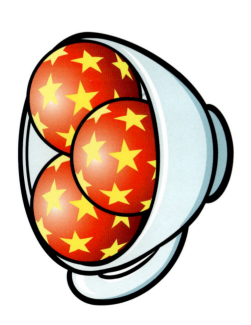
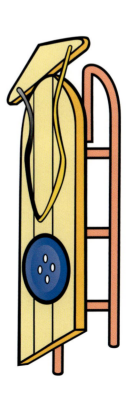

Level 1

Sublevel 7

noun + singular/plural

Example: *Touch the cup with a cat.*

1. Touch the sled with a mitten.

2. Touch the cup with an airplane.

3. Touch the sled with the rings.

4. Touch the hat with a ball.

5. Touch the cup with a cat.

6. Touch the cup with a ring.

7. Touch the hat with a dress.

8. Touch the sled with the airplanes.

Plate 5

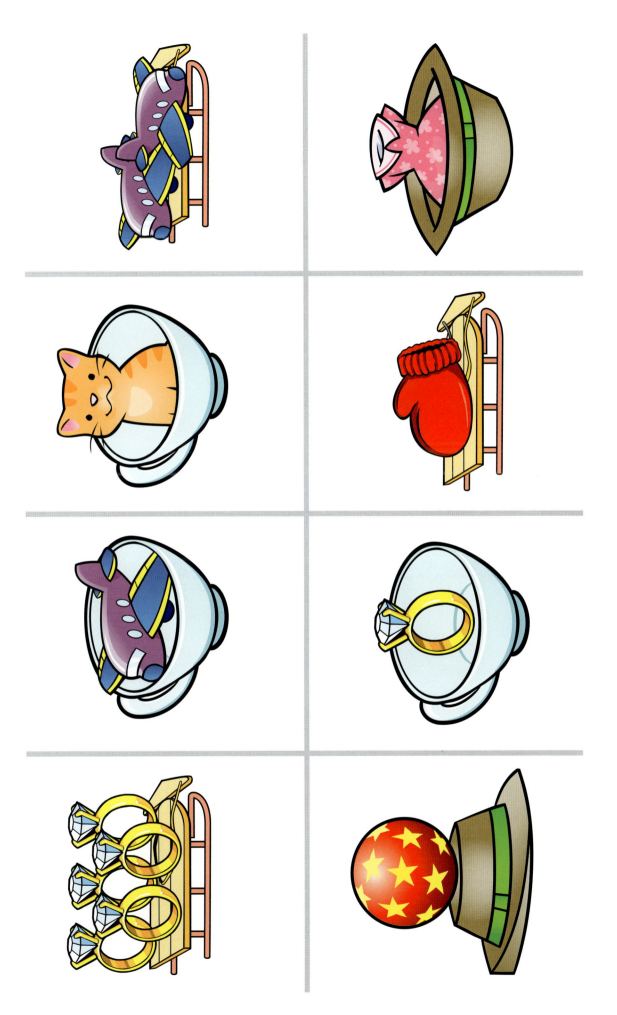

Level 1

Sublevel 7

noun + singular/plural

Example: *Touch the sled with the socks.*

1. Touch the sled with a book.
2. Touch the hat with a button.
3. Touch the cup with a duck.
4. Touch the hat with a sock.
5. Touch the cup with the books.
6. Touch the sled with the socks.
7. Touch the sled with a dog.
8. Touch the hat with a bead.

Plate 6

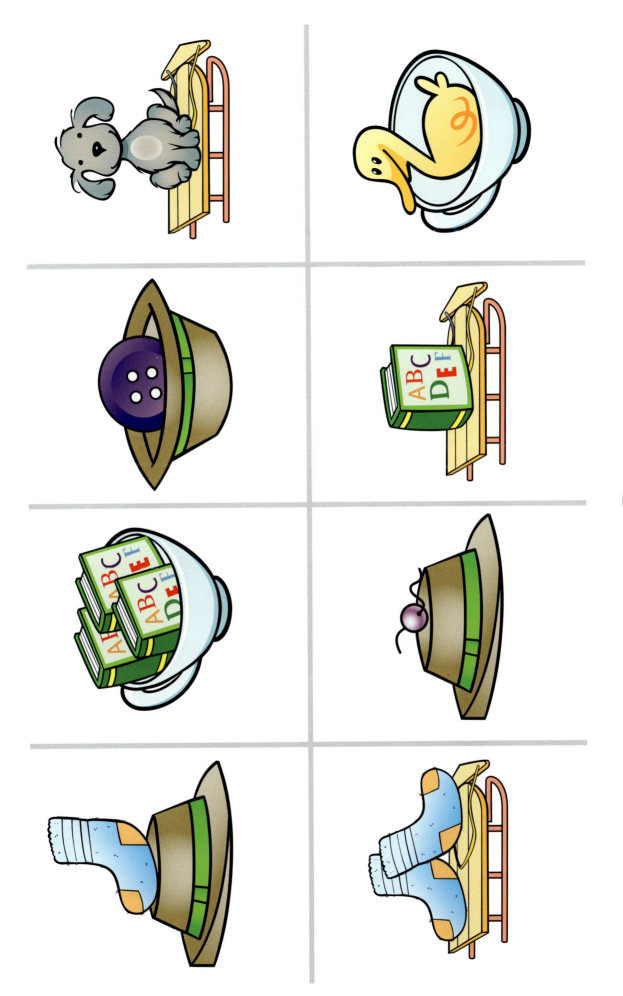

Level 1

Sublevel 7

noun + singular/plural

Example: *Touch the cup with a frog.*

1. Touch the hat with a bear.
2. Touch the hat with a ball.
3. Touch the sled with a bead.
4. Touch the cup with the bears.
5. Touch the sled with a book.
6. Touch the hat with the beads.
7. Touch the cup with a frog.
8. Touch the cup with a dress.

Plate 7

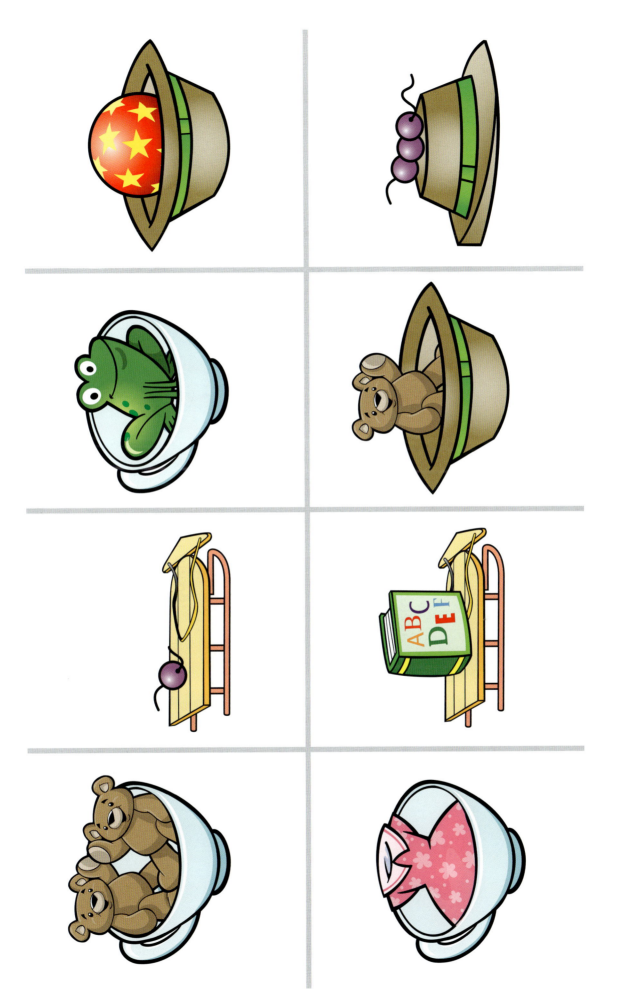

Level 1

Sublevel 7

noun + singular/plural

Example: *Touch the hat with an airplane.*

1. Touch the cup with a frog.
2. Touch the sled with a bead.
3. Touch the cup with a mitten.
4. Touch the hat with the frogs.
5. Touch the hat with a sock.
6. Touch the sled with the mittens.
7. Touch the cup with a book.
8. Touch the hat with an airplane.

Plate 8

©2012 Super Duper® Publications

126

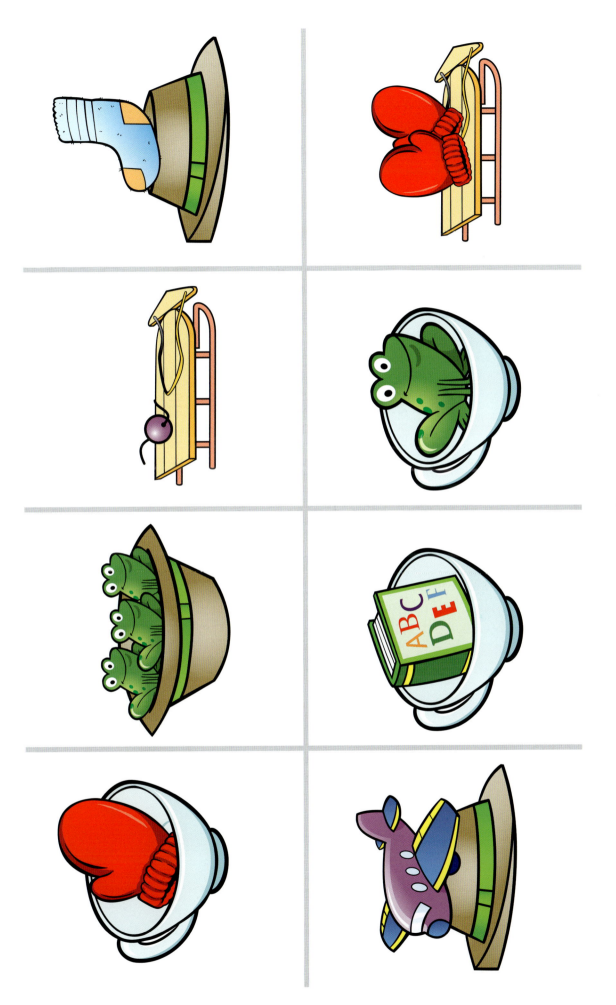

Level 1

Sublevel 8

noun + plural + noun

Example: *Touch the cup with ducks, and touch a bead.*

1. Touch the hat with balls, and touch a duck.

2. Touch the sled with rings, and touch a shoe.

3. Touch the hat with shoes, and touch a ring.

4. Touch the cup with beads, and touch a ball.

5. Touch the cup with ducks, and touch a bead.

6. Touch the sled with rings, and touch a ball.

7. Touch the cup with beads, and touch a duck.

8. Touch the hat with shoes, and touch a shoe.

Plate 1

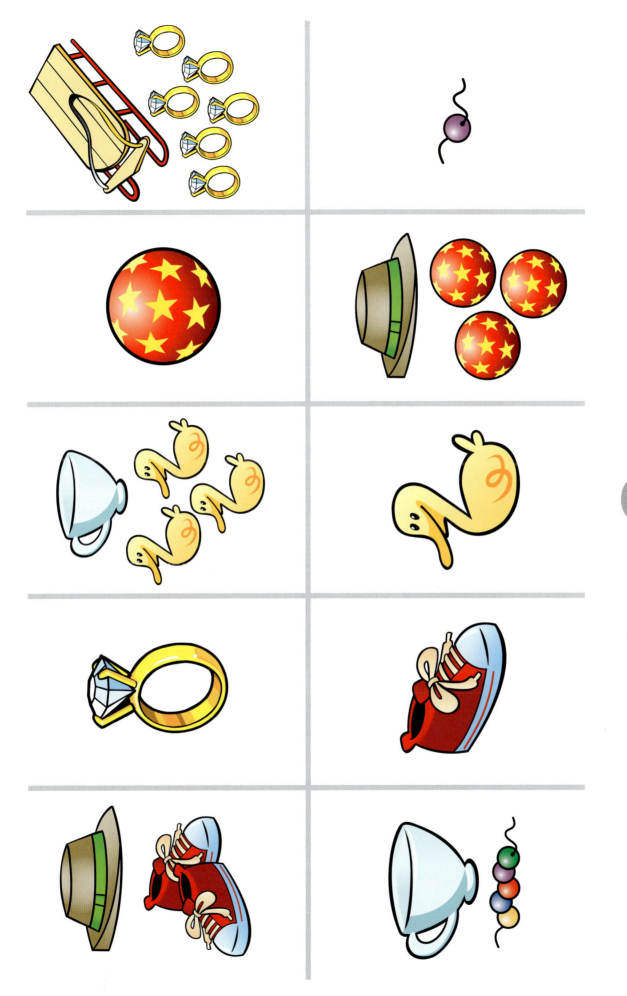

Level 1

Sublevel 8

noun + plural + noun

Example: *Touch the cup with balloons, and touch a ring.*

1. Touch the hat with frogs, and touch a ring.

2. Touch the cup with balloons, and touch a frog.

3. Touch the sled with cups, and touch a ball.

4. Touch the cup with balls, and touch a balloon.

5. Touch the sled with rings, and touch a cup.

6. Touch the cup with balloons, and touch a ring.

7. Touch the hat with frogs, and touch a balloon.

8. Touch the cup with balls, and touch a frog.

©2012 Super Duper® Publications

Plate 2

130

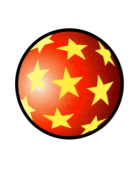
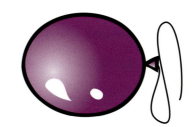
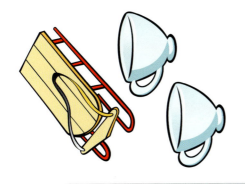
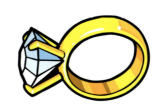

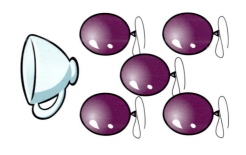
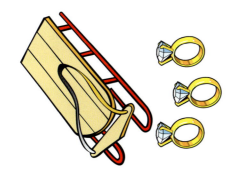
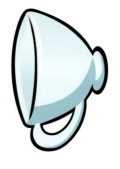
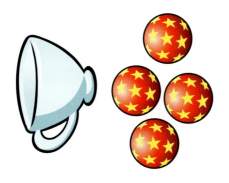
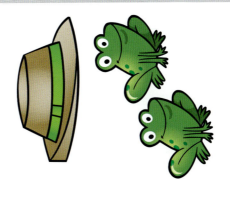

Level 1

Sublevel 8

noun + plural + noun

Example: *Touch the cup with dogs, and touch a duck.*

1. Touch the hat with ducks, and touch a dog.

2. Touch the sled with shoes, and touch a duck.

3. Touch the hat with beads, and touch a ring.

4. Touch a cup with dogs, and touch a bead.

5. Touch the cup with rings, and touch a dog.

6. Touch the hat with ducks, and touch a shoe.

7. Touch the cup with dogs, and touch a duck.

8. Touch the hat with beads, and touch a bead.

Plate 3

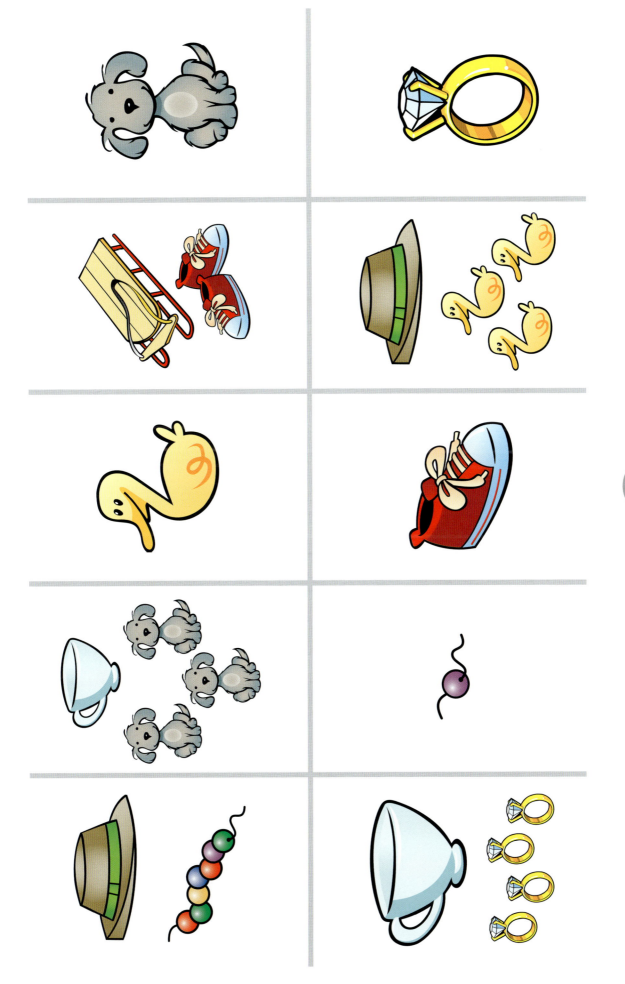

Level 1

Sublevel 8

noun + plural + noun

Example: Touch the cup with balloons, and touch a duck.

1. Touch the hat with frogs, and touch a duck.

2. Touch the sled with cups, and touch a ring.

3. Touch the cup with ducks, and touch a frog.

4. Touch the cup with balloons, and touch a cup.

5. Touch the hat with rings, and touch a balloon.

6. Touch the sled with cups, and touch a frog.

7. Touch the hat with frogs, and touch a ring.

8. Touch the cup with balloons, and touch a duck.

©2012 Super Duper® Publications

Plate 4

134

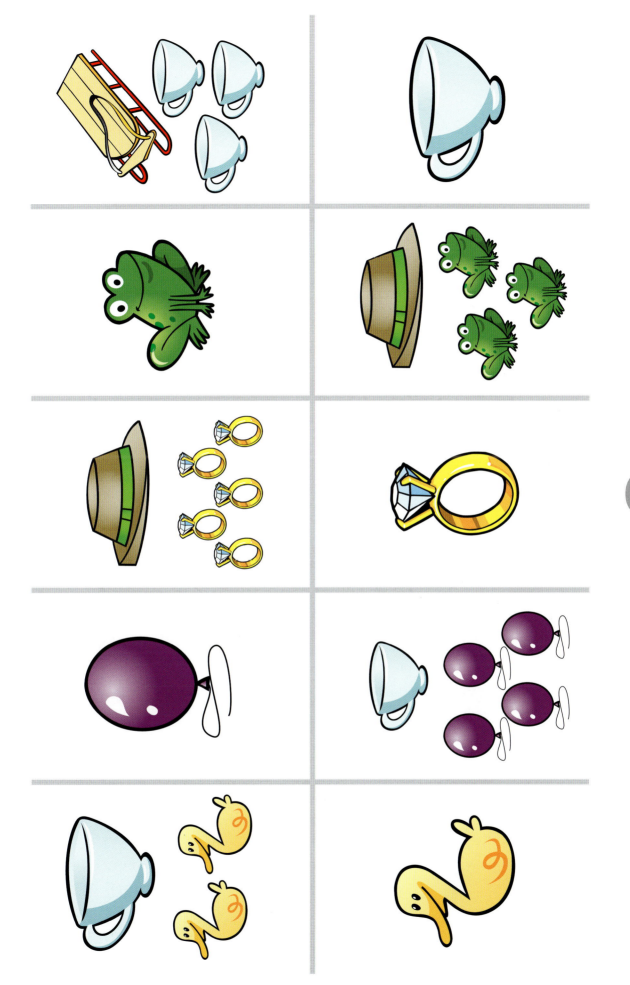

Level 1

Sublevel 9

size + noun

Example: *Touch the big duck.*

1. Touch the big cup.
2. Touch the little dog.
3. Touch the little cup.
4. Touch the little mouse.
5. Touch the big dog.
6. Touch the big bear.
7. Touch the big duck.
8. Touch the big mouse.
9. Touch the little duck.
10. Touch the little bear.

Plate 1

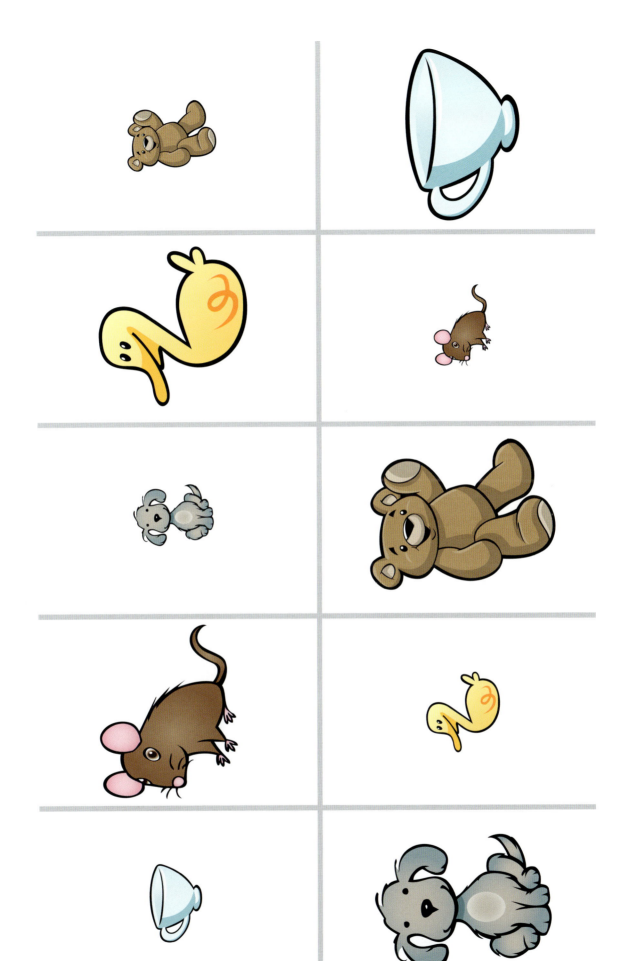

Level 1

Sublevel 9

size + noun

Example: Touch the big frog.

1. Touch the little ball.
2. Touch the big frog.
3. Touch the big book.
4. Touch the big cat.
5. Touch the little book.
6. Touch the big hat.
7. Touch the little cat.
8. Touch the big ball.
9. Touch the little frog.
10. Touch the little hat.

Plate 2

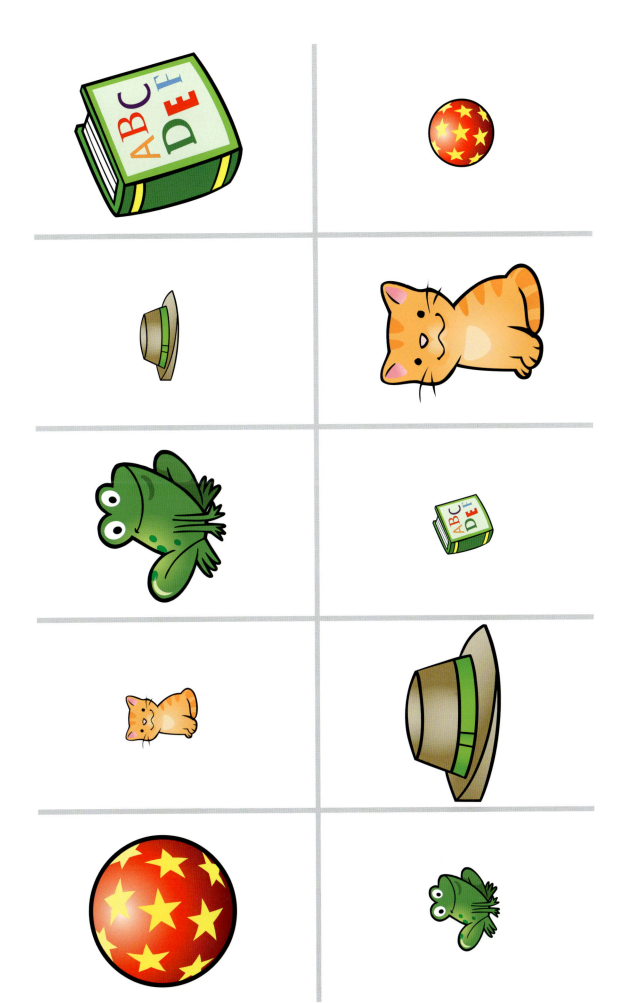

Level 1

Plate 1

Sublevel 10

(size + noun) + (size + noun)

Example: *Touch the little cat with little shoes.*

1. Touch the big cat with big shoes.

2. Touch the little cat with big shoes.

3. Touch the big cat with little shoes.

4. Touch the little cat with little shoes.

©2012 Super Duper® Publications

140

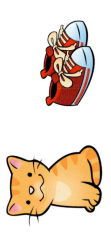
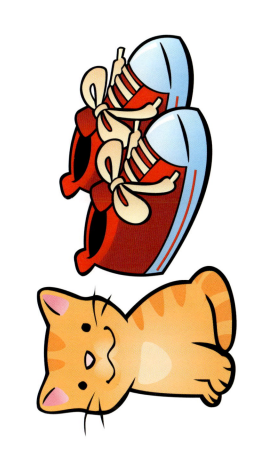

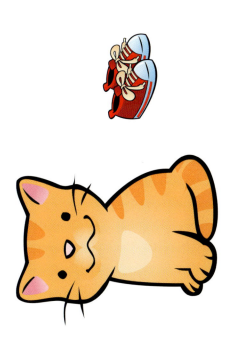
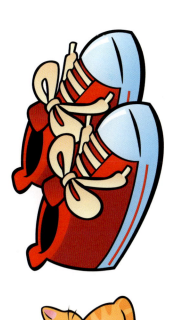
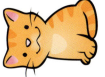

Level 1

Sublevel 10

(size + noun) + (size + noun)

Example: *Touch the big mouse with a little dress.*

1. Touch the little mouse with a little dress.

2. Touch the big mouse with a little dress.

3. Touch the little mouse with a big dress.

4. Touch the big mouse with a big dress.

Plate 2

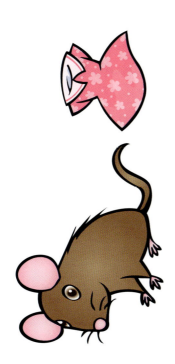
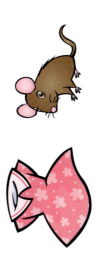

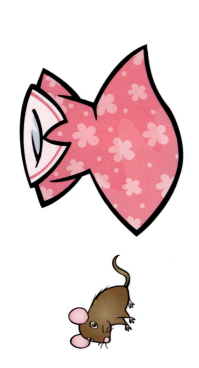
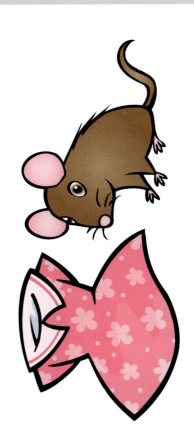

Level 1

Sublevel 10

(size + noun) + (size + noun)

Example: *Touch the little dog with a big sock.*

1. Touch the big dog with a big sock.
2. Touch the little dog with a big mitten.
3. Touch the little dog with a big mitten.
4. Touch the big dog with a little sock.
5. Touch the big dog with a little mitten.
6. Touch the little dog with a little sock.
7. Touch the little dog with a little mitten.
8. Touch the big dog with a big mitten.

Plate 3

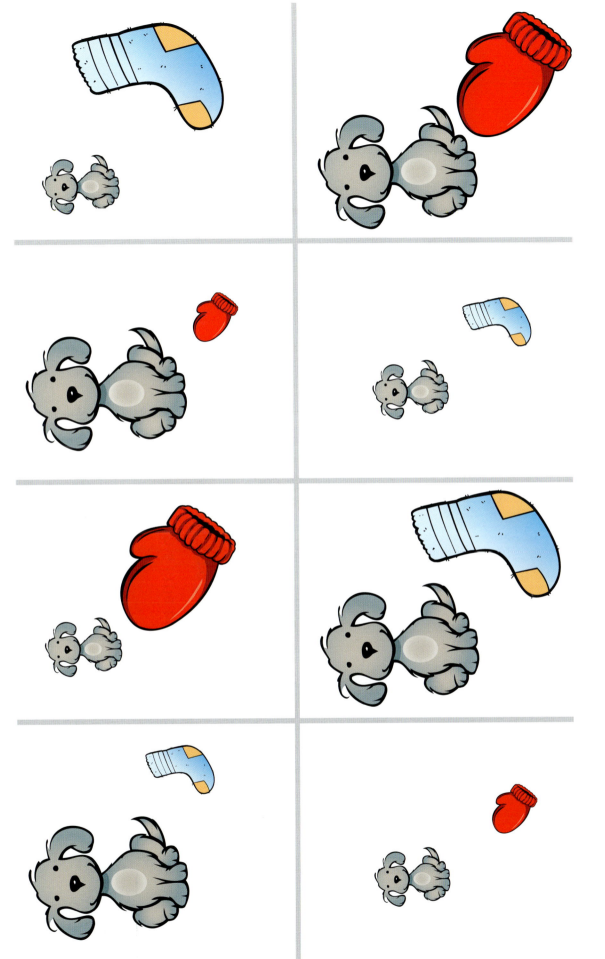

Level 1

Sublevel 10

(size + noun) + (size + noun)

Example: *Touch the little bear with a little ball.*

1. Touch the little bear with a little book.

2. Touch the big bear with a big book.

3. Touch the little bear with a big ball.

4. Touch the big bear with a big ball.

5. Touch the big bear with a little book.

6. Touch the little bear with a big book.

7. Touch the big bear with a little ball.

8. Touch the little bear with a little ball.

Plate 4

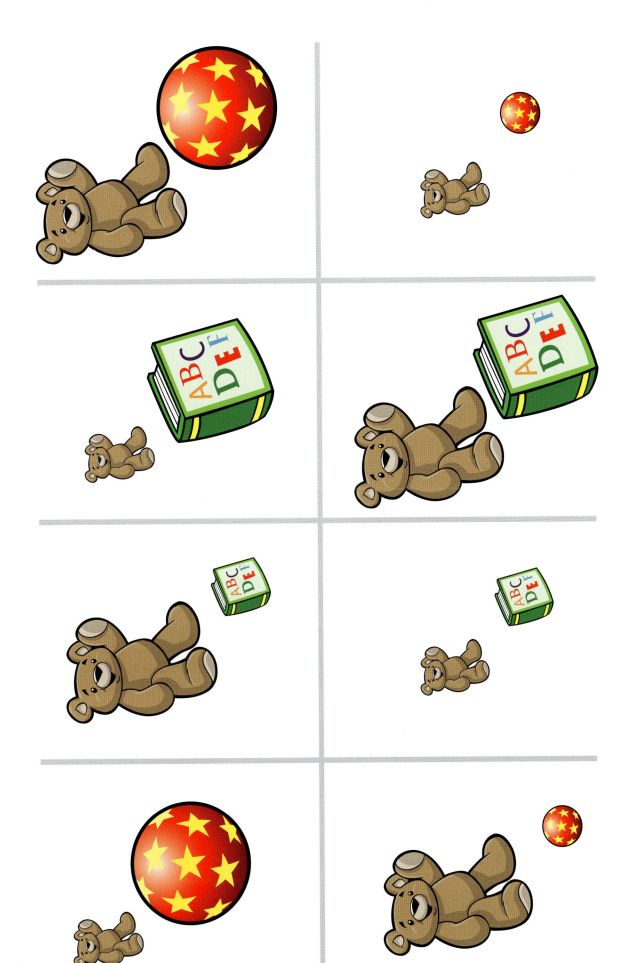

Level 1

Plate 1

Sublevel 11

noun + (size + singular/plural)

Example: *Touch the sled with the little dogs.*

1. Touch the sled with the little dogs.

2. Touch the sled with a big dog.

3. Touch the sled with the big dogs.

4. Touch the sled with a little dog.

©2012 Super Duper® Publications

148

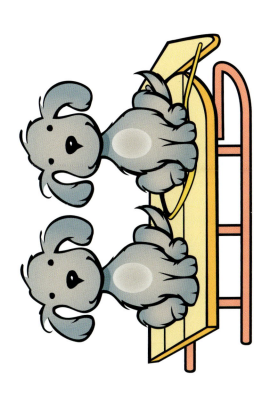
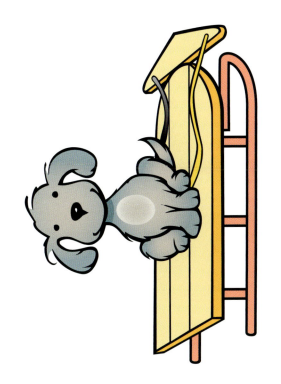

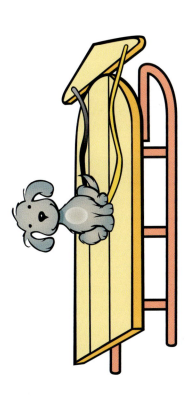
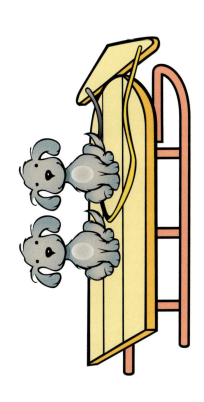

Level 1

Sublevel 11

noun + (size + singular/plural)

Example: *Touch the dress with the big buttons.*

1. Touch the dress with a little button.

2. Touch the dress with the big buttons.

3. Touch the dress with the little buttons.

4. Touch the dress with a big button.

Plate 2

©2012 Super Duper® Publications

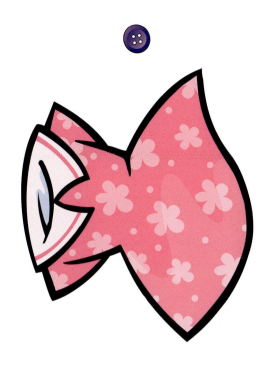
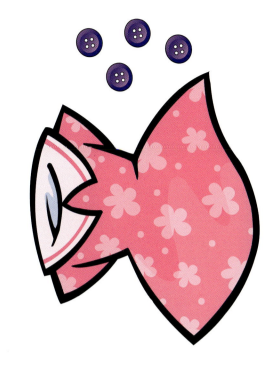
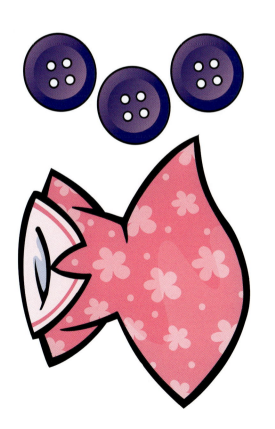
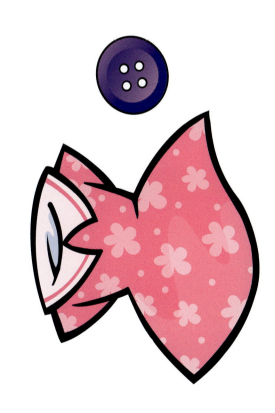

Level 1

Sublevel 11

noun + (size + singular/plural)

Example: *Touch the cup with the big beads.*

1. Touch the cup with the little beads.
2. Touch the cup with a big bead.
3. Touch the cup with the big beads.
4. Touch the cup with a little bead.

Plate 3

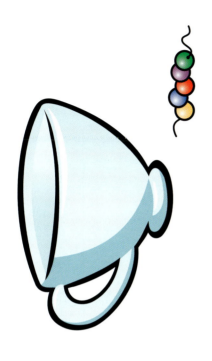
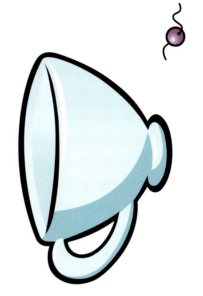
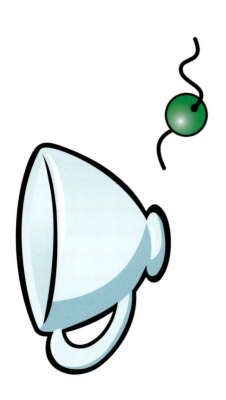
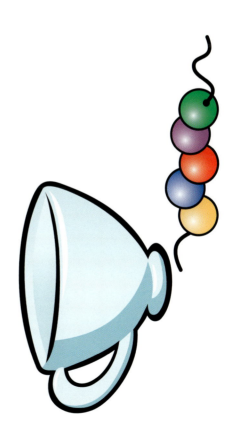

Level 1

Sublevel 11

noun + (size + singular/plural)

Example: Touch the hat with the big frogs.

1. Touch the hat with a little frog.

2. Touch the hat with a big frog.

3. Touch the hat with the little frogs.

4. Touch the hat with the big frogs.

Plate 4

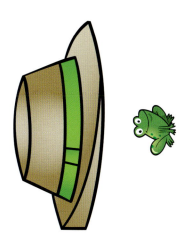
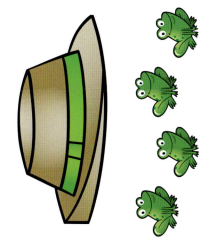
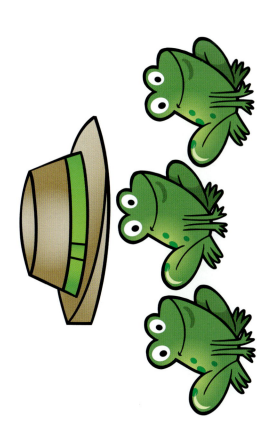
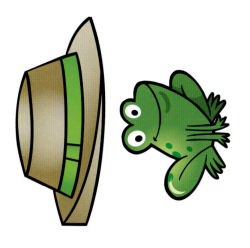

Level 1

Sublevel 12

noun + (size + singular/plural) + noun + (size + singular/plural)

Example: *Touch the sled with the little cats and the sled with a big duck.*

1. Touch the sled with the little cats and the sled with a big duck.
2. Touch the sled with a big cat and the sled with the little ducks.
3. Touch the sled with a big duck and the sled with a big cat.
4. Touch the sled with the little ducks and the sled with the little cats.

Plate 1

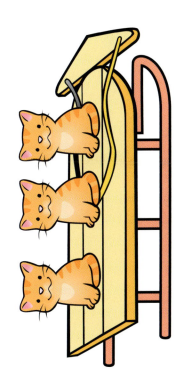
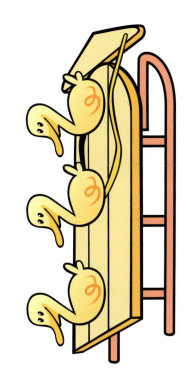

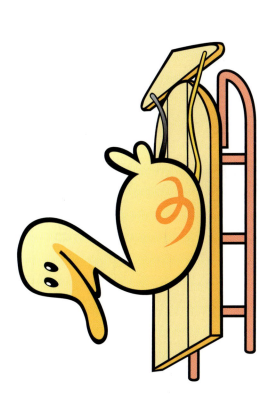
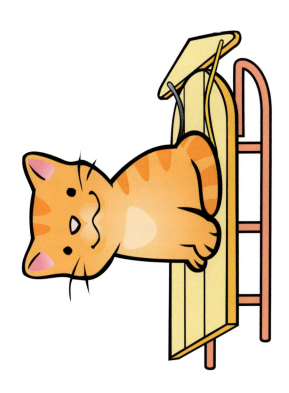

Level 1

Sublevel 12

noun + (size + singular/plural) + noun + (size + singular/plural)

Example: *Touch the cup with the little balloons and the cup with the little beads.*

1. Touch the cup with a big balloon and the cup with a big bead.
2. Touch the cup with the little balloons and the cup with the little beads.
3. Touch the cup with a big bead and the cup with the little balloons.
4. Touch the cup with the little beads and the cup with a big balloon.

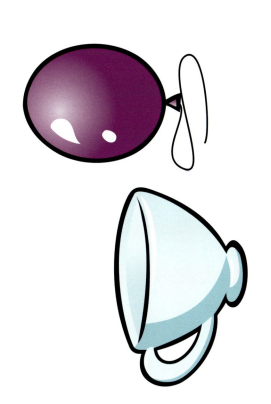
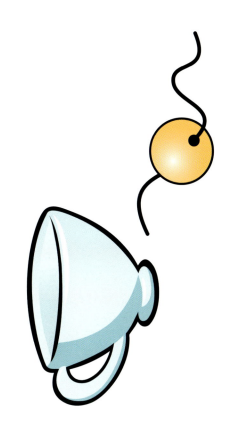
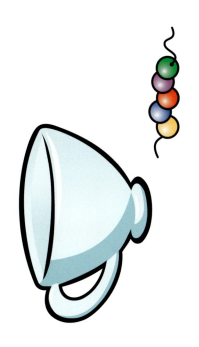
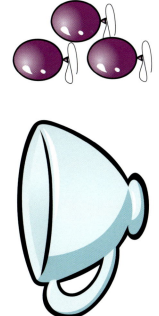

Level 1

Sublevel 12

noun + (size + singular/plural) + noun + (size + singular/plural)

Example: Touch the cup with the big rings and the frog with the big shoes.

1. Touch the hat with a big dog and the cup with the big rings.

2. Touch the frog with the little shoes and the sled with a big cat.

3. Touch the frog with the big shoes and the cup with a little ring.

4. Touch the sled with the little cats and the hat with the little dogs.

5. Touch the cup with a little ring and the hat with a big dog.

6. Touch the sled with a big cat and the frog with the little shoes.

7. Touch the cup with the big rings and the frog with the big shoes.

8. Touch the hat with the little dogs and the sled with the little cats.

Plate 3

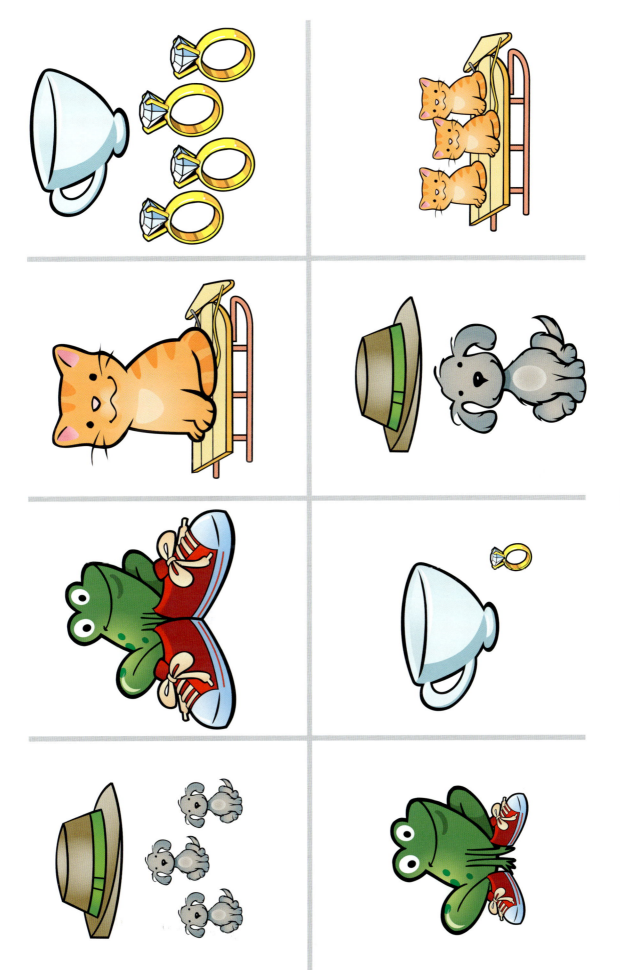

Level 1

Sublevel 12

noun + (size + singular/plural) + noun + (size + singular/plural)

Example: Touch the hat with the big bears and the dog with the little mittens.

1. Touch the hat with a little bear and the cup with the big frogs.

2. Touch the sled with a big book and the dog with the big mittens.

3. Touch the cup with a little frog and the hat with the big bears.

4. Touch the dog with the little mittens and the sled with the little books.

5. Touch the dog with the big mittens and the hat with a little bear.

6. Touch the sled with little books and the cup with a little frog.

7. Touch the cup with the big frogs and the sled with a big book.

8. Touch the hat with the big bears and the dog with the little mittens.

Plate 4

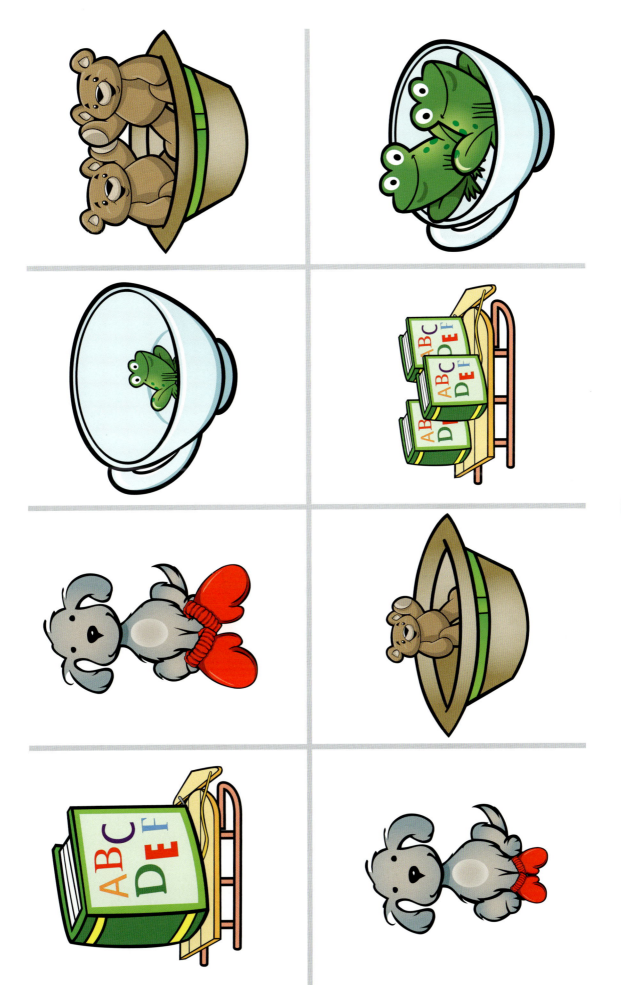

Level 1

Sublevel 13

color + noun

Example: *Touch the green shoe.*

1. Touch the green shoe.
2. Touch the yellow mitten.
3. Touch the blue shoe.
4. Touch the red mitten.

©2012 Super Duper® Publications

Plate 1

164

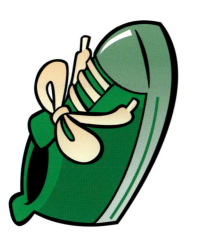
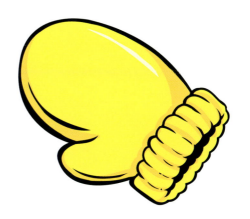
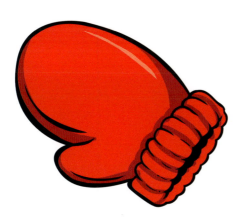
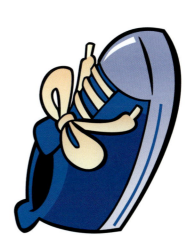

Level 1

Sublevel 13

color + noun

Example: *Touch the red airplane.*

1. Touch the blue mitten.
2. Touch the red airplane.
3. Touch the green mitten.
4. Touch the yellow airplane.

Plate 2

©2012 Super Duper® Publications

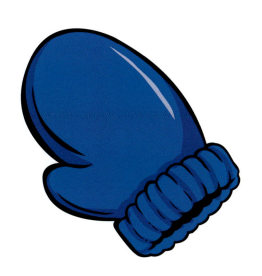
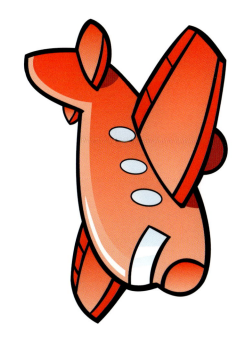
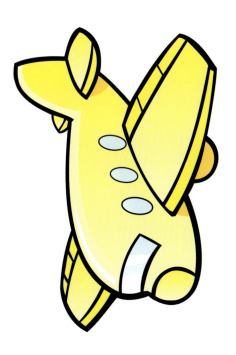
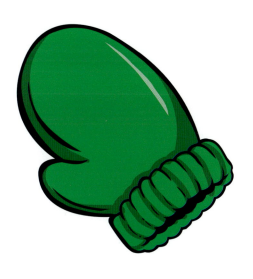
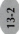

Level 1

Sublevel 13

color + noun

Example: Touch the red mitten.

1. Touch the yellow airplane.
2. Touch the blue mitten.
3. Touch the yellow shoe.
4. Touch the blue airplane.
5. Touch the red shoe.
6. Touch the green mitten.
7. Touch the red mitten.
8. Touch the green shoe.

Plate 3

©2012 Super Duper® Publications

168

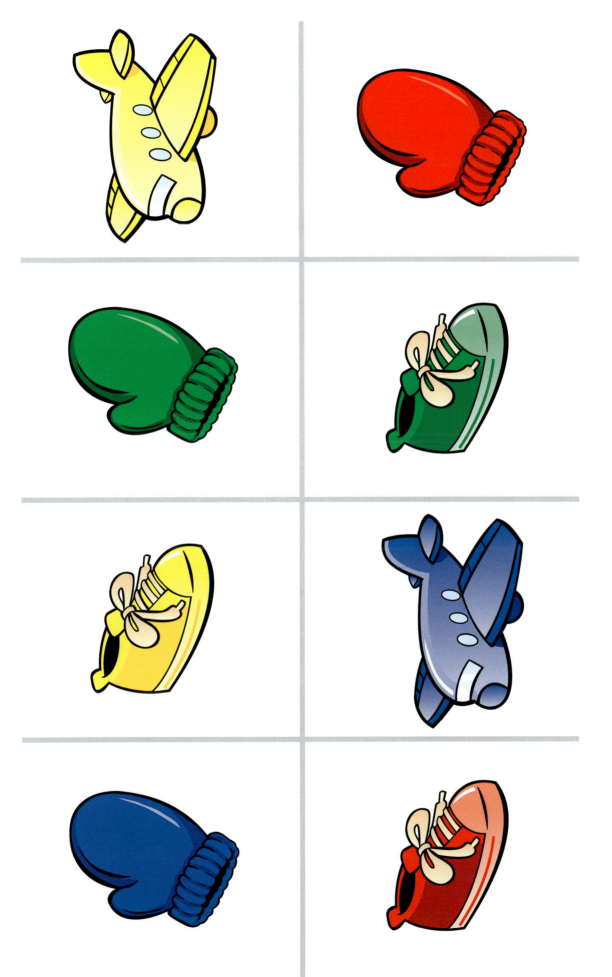

Level 1

Sublevel 13

color + noun

Example: *Touch the red balloon.*

1. Touch the yellow book.
2. Touch the green balloon.
3. Touch the blue book.
4. Touch the blue balloon.
5. Touch the red book.
6. Touch the red airplane.
7. Touch the green airplane.
8. Touch the red balloon.

Plate 4

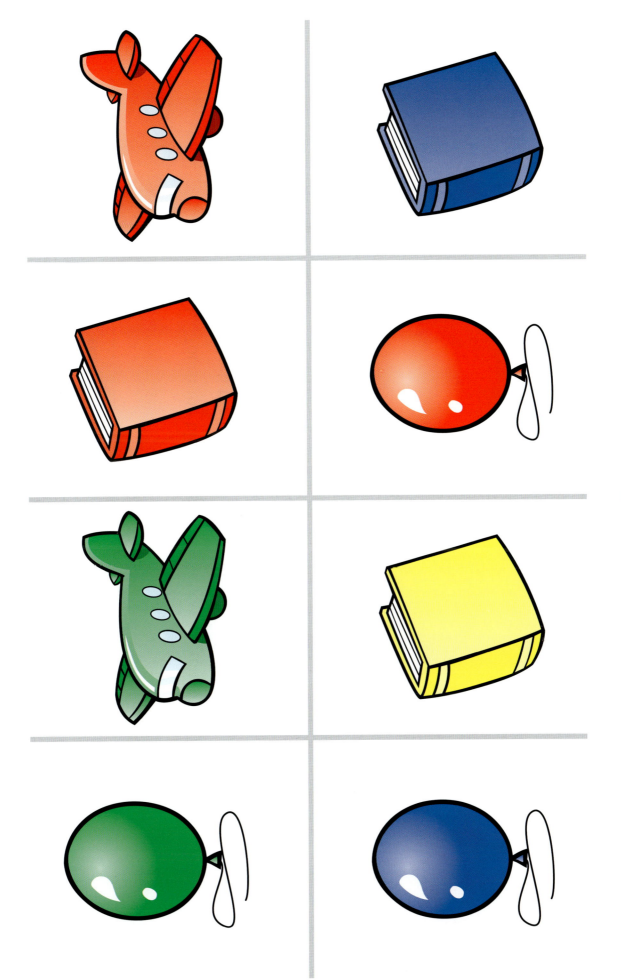

Level 1

Sublevel 14

(color + noun) + (color + noun)

Example: Touch the red dress with a yellow button.

1. Touch the blue dress with a yellow button.
2. Touch the red dress with a green button.
3. Touch the green dress with a blue button.
4. Touch the yellow dress with a green button.
5. Touch the blue dress with a red button.
6. Touch the red dress with a yellow button.

Plate 1

©2012 Super Duper® Publications

172

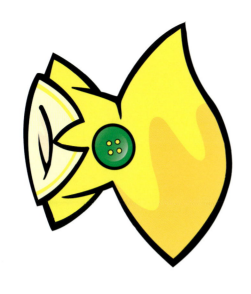
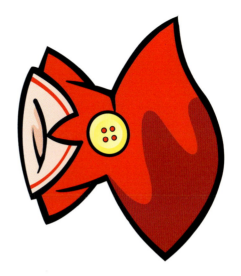
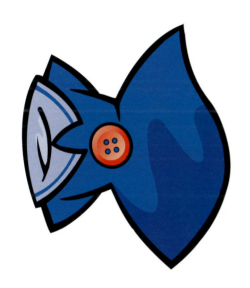
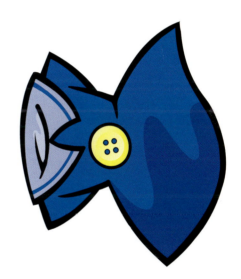
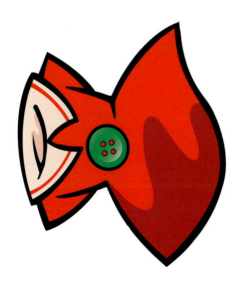
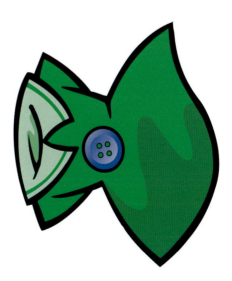

Level 1

Sublevel 14

(color + noun) + (color + noun)

Example: Touch the green frog with a blue shoe.

1. Touch the blue frog with a red sock.

2. Touch the green cat with a red shoe.

3. Touch the green frog with a blue shoe.

4. Touch the yellow cat with a green sock.

5. Touch the yellow cat with a blue sock.

6. Touch the red frog with a yellow shoe.

Plate 2

©2012 Super Duper® Publications

1174

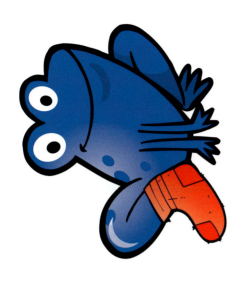
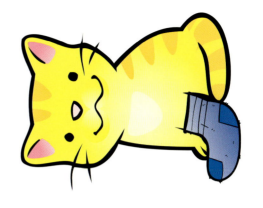
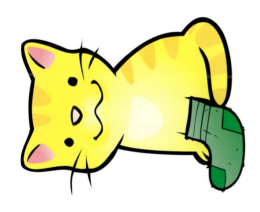
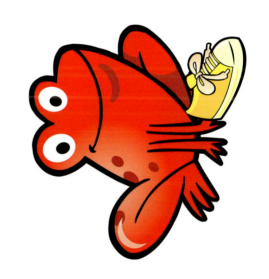
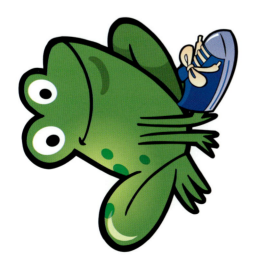
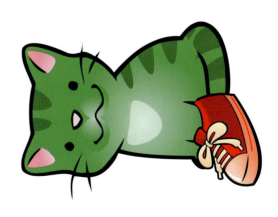

Level 1

Sublevel 14

(color + noun) + (color + noun)

Example: *Touch the red bear with a blue mitten.*

1. Touch the yellow bear with a red mitten.
2. Touch the red bear with a green mitten.
3. Touch the green bear with a red mitten.
4. Touch the red bear with a blue mitten.
5. Touch the yellow bear with a blue mitten.
6. Touch the blue bear with a green mitten.

©2012 Super Duper® Publications

Plate 3

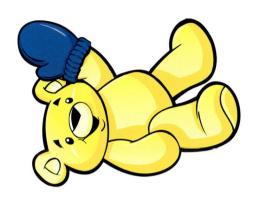
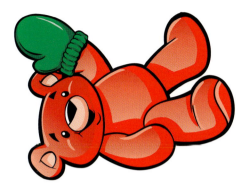
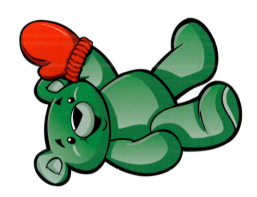
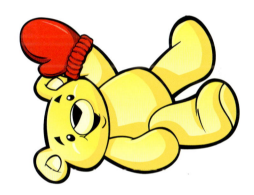
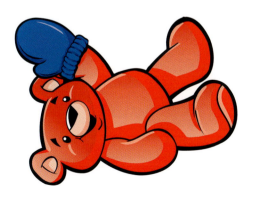
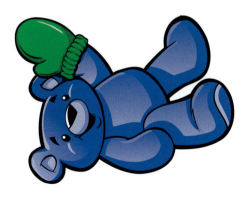

Level 1

Sublevel 14

(color + noun) + (color + noun)

Example: *Touch the blue sled with a green bead.*

1. Touch the red cup with a yellow bead.
2. Touch the blue cup with a yellow bead.
3. Touch the red sled with a green bead.
4. Touch the yellow cup with a red bead.
5. Touch the blue sled with a green bead.
6. Touch the green sled with a blue bead.

Plate 4

©2012 Super Duper® Publications

178

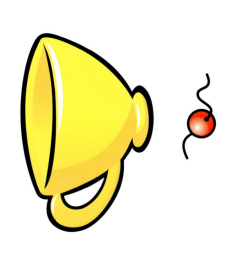
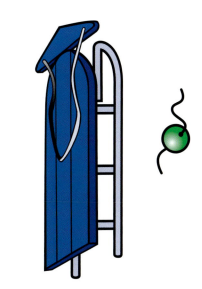
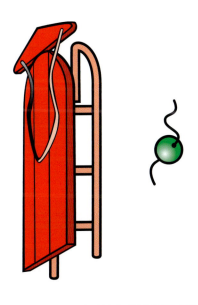
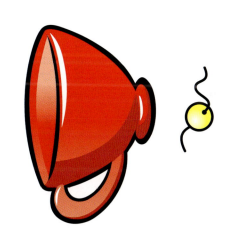
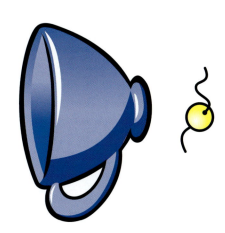
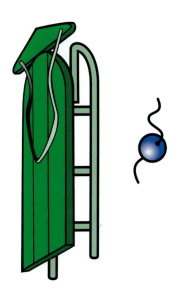

Level 1

Sublevel 15

(color + noun) + (color + singular/plural)

Example: *Touch the blue frog with the green balloons.*

1. Touch the green frog with a red balloon.

2. Touch the blue frog with a green balloon.

3. Touch the red frog with the yellow balloons.

4. Touch the yellow frog with a blue balloon.

5. Touch the blue frog with the green balloons.

6. Touch the blue frog with a yellow balloon.

7. Touch the red frog with the blue balloons.

8. Touch the green frog with the red balloons.

Plate 1

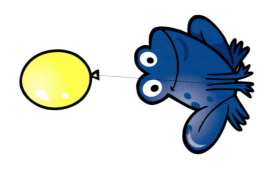
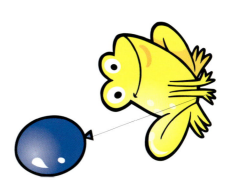
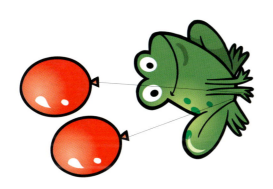
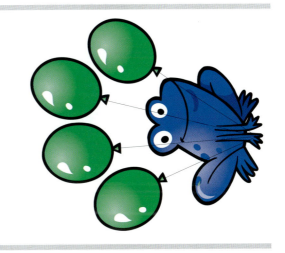
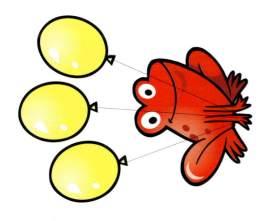
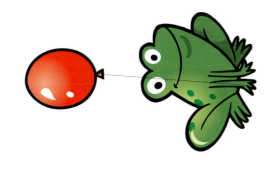
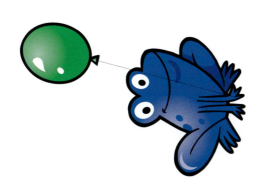
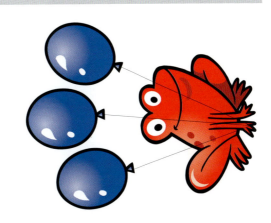

15-1

Level 1

Sublevel 15

(color + noun) + (color + singular/plural)

Example: Touch the red bear with a yellow book.

1. Touch the red bear with a green book.

2. Touch the green bear with a blue book.

3. Touch the blue bear with the yellow books.

4. Touch the yellow bear with a red book.

5. Touch the blue bear with the green books.

6. Touch the red bear with a yellow book.

7. Touch the yellow bear with the red books.

8. Touch the green bear with the blue books.

Plate 2

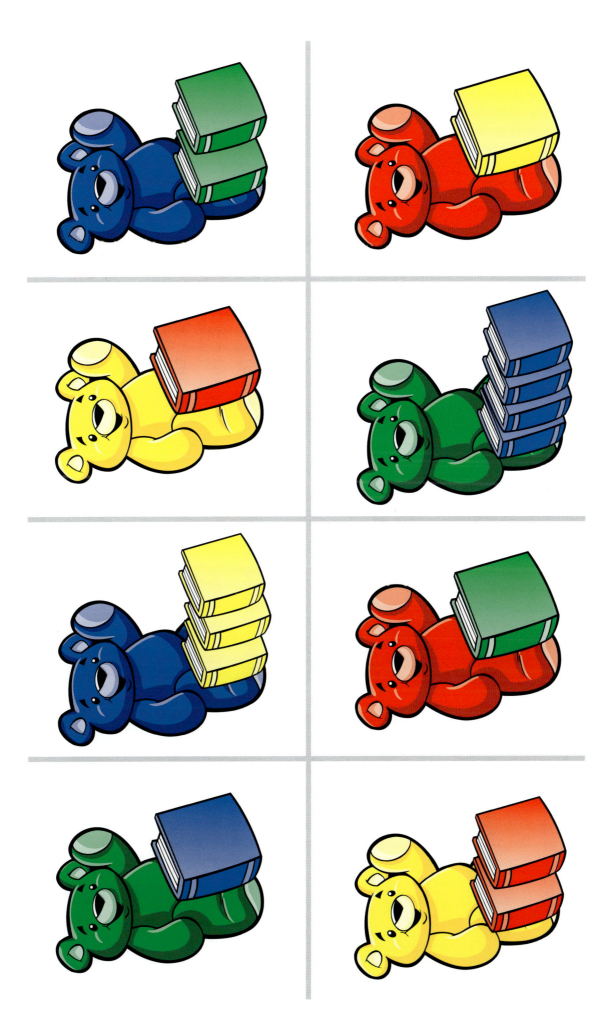

Level 1

Sublevel 15

(color + noun) + (color + singular/plural)

Example: Touch the yellow cup with the green beads.

1. Touch the blue cup with a red bead.

2. Touch the red cup with the blue beads.

3. Touch the red cup with the yellow beads.

4. Touch the blue cup with a green bead.

5. Touch the green cup with the red beads.

6. Touch the yellow cup with a blue bead.

7. Touch the yellow cup with the green beads.

8. Touch the green cup with a yellow bead.

Plate 3

©2012 Super Duper® Publications

184

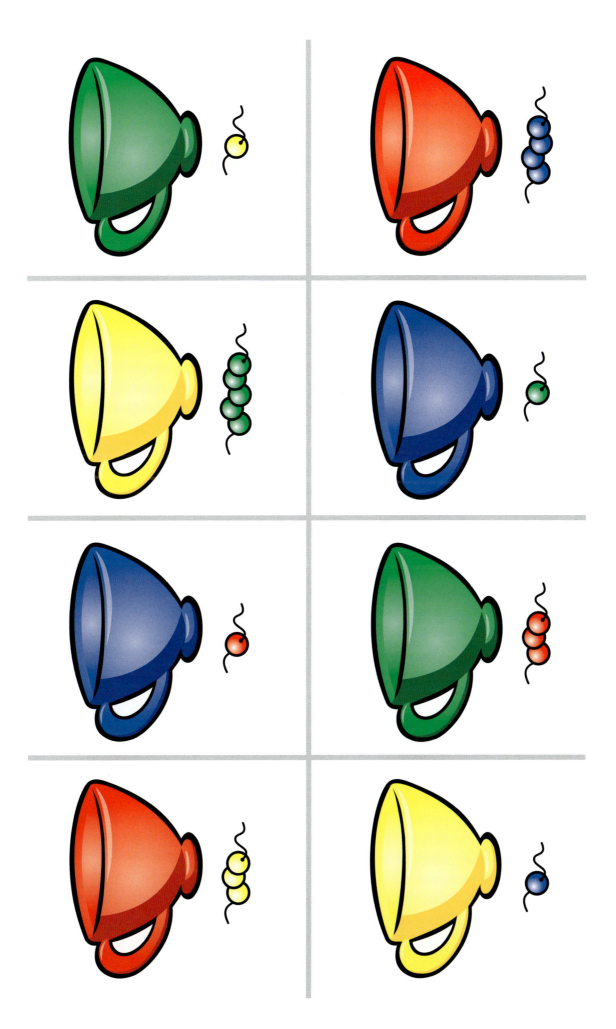

Level 1

Sublevel 15

(color + noun) + (color + singular/plural)

Example: *Touch the blue hat with a yellow ball.*

1. Touch the blue hat with the yellow balls.
2. Touch the red hat with the blue balls.
3. Touch the green hat with a blue ball.
4. Touch the yellow hat with the red balls.
5. Touch the red hat with a green ball.
6. Touch the yellow hat with the green balls.
7. Touch the green hat with a red ball.
8. Touch the blue hat with a yellow ball.

Plate 4

©2012 Super Duper® Publications

186

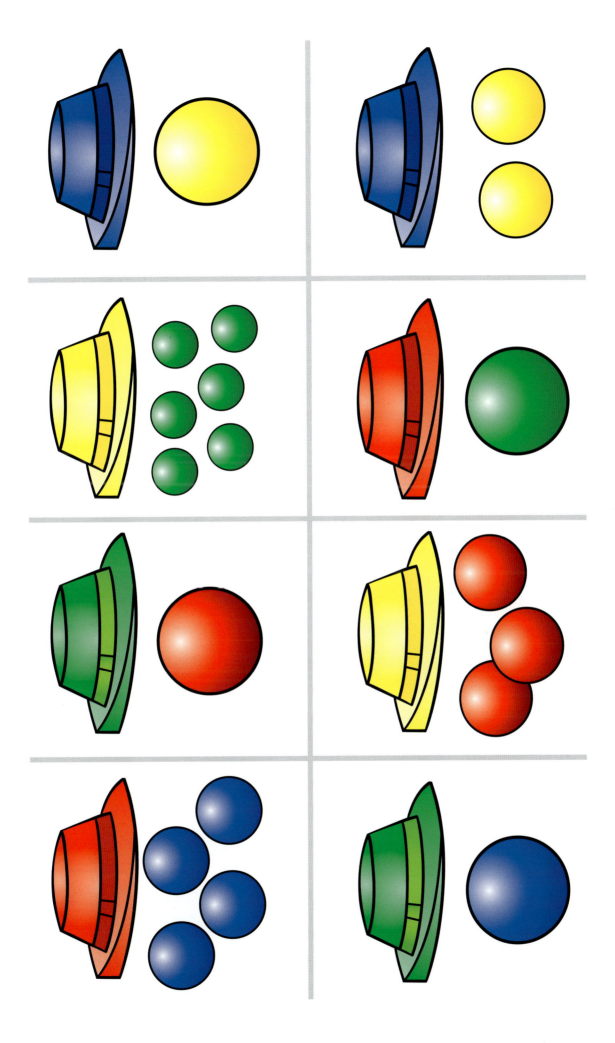

Level 1

Sublevel 16

(color + singular/plural) + (color + singular/plural)

Example: Touch a green ball and the red buttons.

1. Touch the green socks and a red bead.

2. Touch a red sock and the blue beads.

3. Touch the blue balls and a yellow button.

4. Touch a green ball and the red buttons.

5. Touch the blue beads and a green ball.

6. Touch a red bead and the blue balls.

7. Touch the green socks and a yellow button.

8. Touch a red sock and the red buttons.

Plate 1

©2012 Super Duper® Publications

188

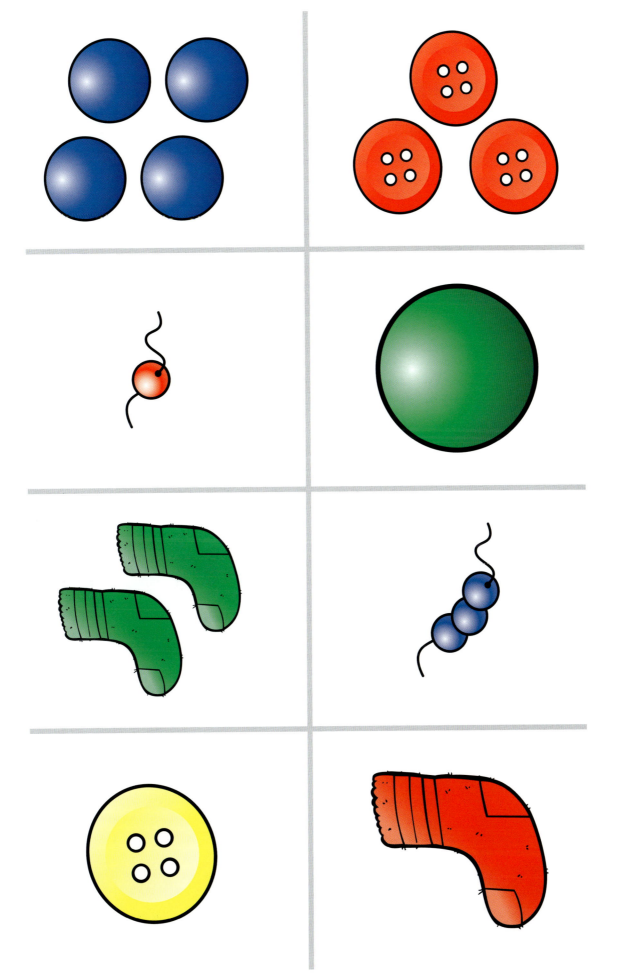

Level 1

Plate 2

Sublevel 16

(color + singular/plural) + (color + singular/plural)

Example: Touch a blue shoe and the red shoes.

1. Touch the red hats and a blue shoe.

2. Touch a yellow ring and the yellow balloons.

3. Touch the red shoes and a blue hat.

4. Touch a green balloon and the yellow balloons.

5. Touch a blue shoe and the red shoes.

6. Touch the green rings and a yellow ring.

7. Touch a blue hat and the red hats.

8. Touch the green rings and a green balloon.

©2012 Super Duper® Publications

190

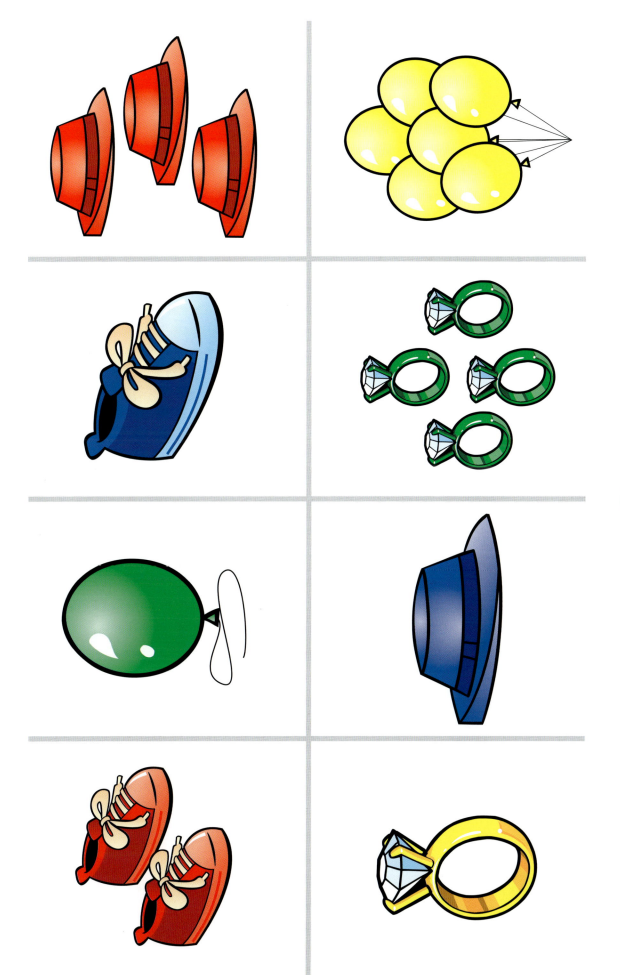

Level 1

Sublevel 16

(color + singular/plural) + (color + singular/plural)

Example: *Touch a blue cat and the yellow dogs.*

1. Touch a green dog and the blue dresses.
2. Touch the red cups and a blue cat.
3. Touch a blue cup and the yellow cats.
4. Touch the yellow dogs and a green dress.
5. Touch the yellow cats and a green dog.
6. Touch a blue cat and the yellow dogs.
7. Touch the blue dresses and a blue cup.
8. Touch a green dress and the red cups.

Plate 3

©2012 Super Duper® Publications

192

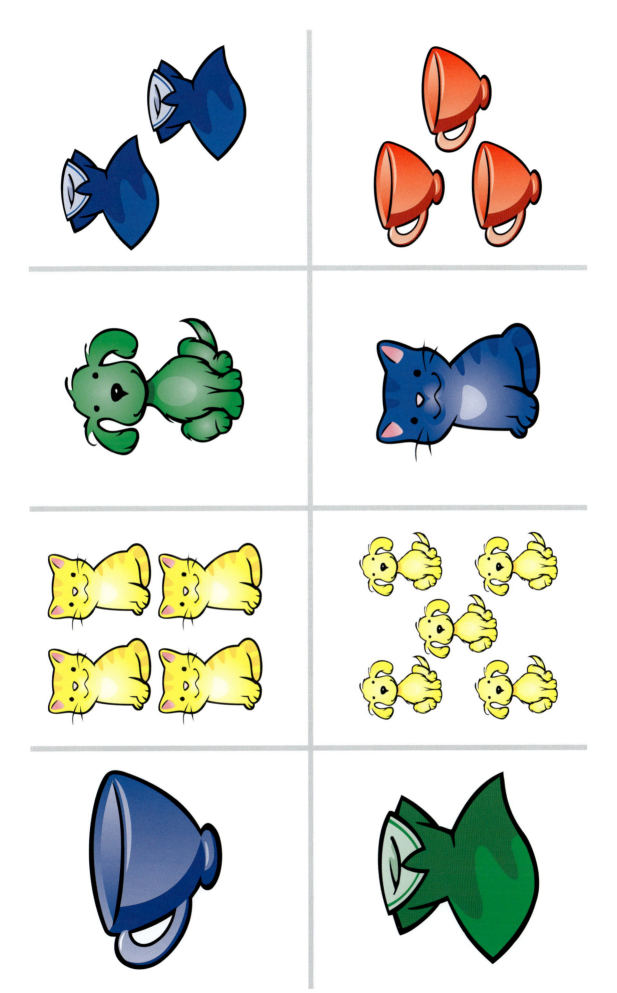

Level 1

Sublevel 16

(color + singular/plural) + (color + singular/plural)

Example: Touch a green mitten and the green airplanes.

1. Touch the blue books and a green mitten.

2. Touch the yellow ducks and a blue airplane.

3. Touch a red book and the yellow mittens.

4. Touch a red duck and the green airplanes.

5. Touch the yellow mittens and a blue airplane.

6. Touch a red book and the yellow ducks.

7. Touch a green mitten and the green airplanes.

8. Touch the blue books and a red duck.

©2012 Super Duper® Publications

Plate 4

194

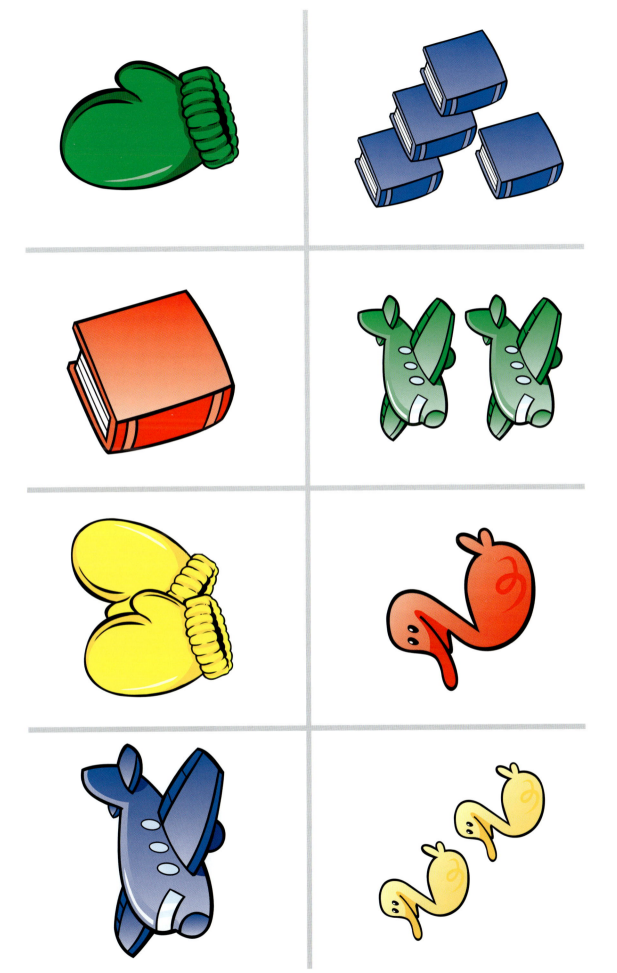

Level 1

Sublevel 17

size + color + noun

Example: *Touch the big, green sock.*

1. Touch the little, blue sock.
2. Touch the little, red sock.
3. Touch the big, green book.
4. Touch the big, green sock.
5. Touch the little, blue book.
6. Touch the big, red book.

Plate 1

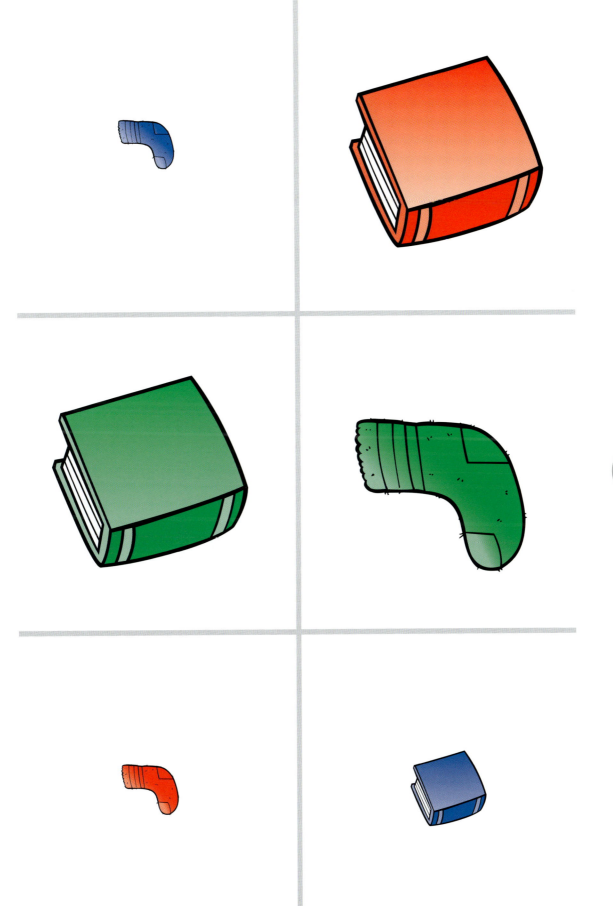

Level 1

Sublevel 17

size + color + noun

Example: *Touch the big, red ring.*

1. Touch the little, yellow mouse.
2. Touch the little, red mouse.
3. Touch the little, blue ring.
4. Touch the big, green mouse.
5. Touch the big, red ring.
6. Touch the big, green ring.

Plate 2

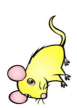
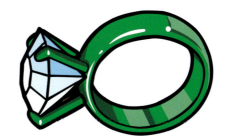
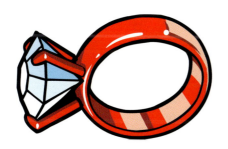
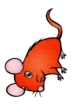

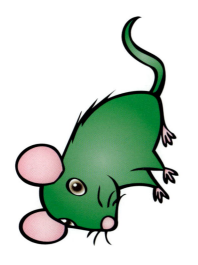

Level 1

Sublevel 17

size + color + noun

Example: *Touch the big, red airplane.*

1. Touch the little, red bear.
2. Touch the little, green airplane.
3. Touch the big, blue bear.
4. Touch the big, yellow airplane.
5. Touch the little, yellow bear.
6. Touch the big, red airplane.

Plate 3

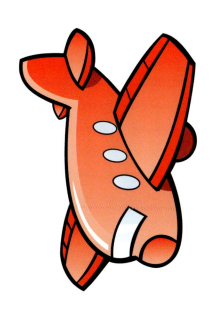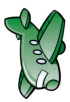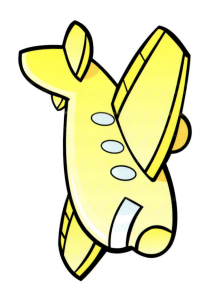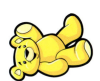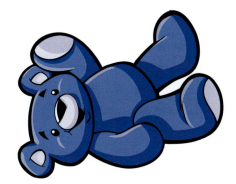

Level 1

Sublevel 18

noun + (size + color + singular/plural)

Example: *Touch the dog with little, red balloon.*

1. Touch the dog with a big, blue balloon.

2. Touch the dog with a big, yellow balloon.

3. Touch the dog with a little, red balloon.

4. Touch the dog with a big, green balloon.

5. Touch the dog with a little, blue balloon.

6. Touch the dog with a little, yellow balloon.

Plate 1

©2012 Super Duper® Publications

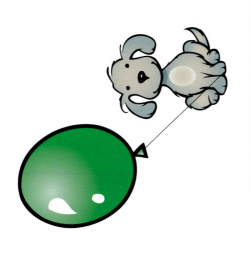
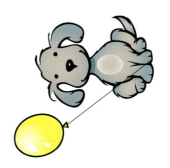
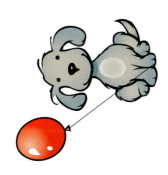
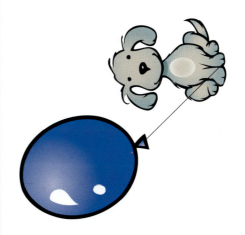

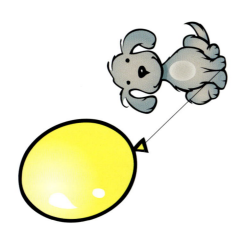
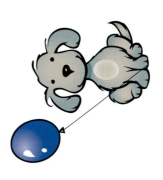

Level 1

Sublevel 18

noun + (size + color + singular/plural)

Example: Touch the duck with little, green shoes.

1. Touch the duck with big, green shoes.
2. Touch the duck with little, yellow shoes.
3. Touch the duck with big, red shoes.
4. Touch the duck with little, blue shoes.
5. Touch the duck with big, yellow shoes.
6. Touch the duck with little, green shoes.

Plate 2

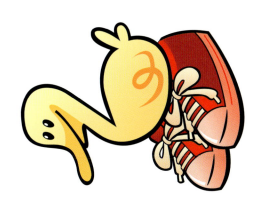
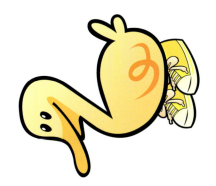
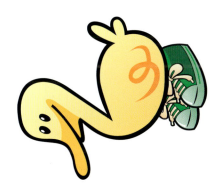
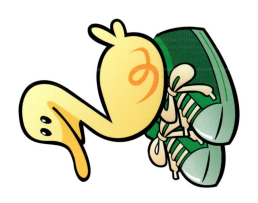
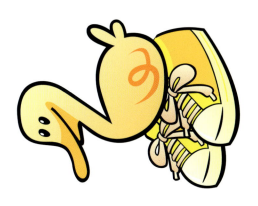
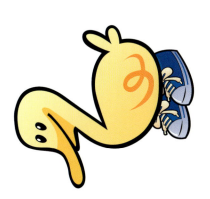
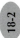

Level 1

Sublevel 18

noun + (size + color + singular/plural)

Example: Touch the frog with little, red mittens.

1. Touch the frog with big, green mittens.
2. Touch the frog with little, red mittens.
3. Touch the frog with big, blue mittens.
4. Touch the frog with little, yellow mittens.
5. Touch the frog with little, blue mittens.
6. Touch the frog with big, yellow mittens.

Plate 3

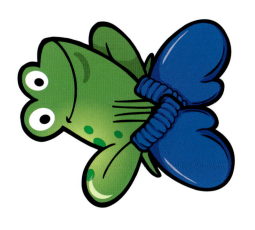
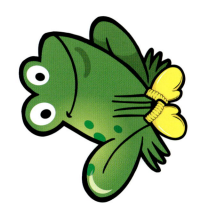
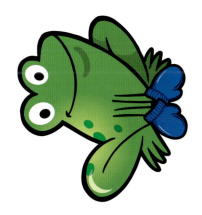
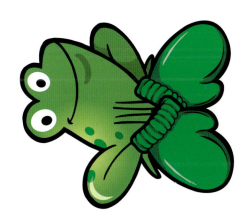
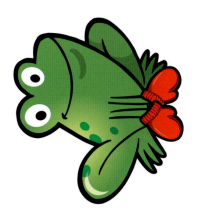
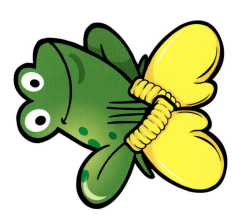

Level 1

Sublevel 18

noun + (size + color + singular/plural)

Example: *Touch the duck with the little, red balls.*

1. Touch the duck with a big, red ball.
2. Touch the duck with a big, blue ball.
3. Touch the duck with the little, red balls.
4. Touch the duck with a little, green ball.
5. Touch the duck with the big, yellow balls.
6. Touch the duck with a little, blue ball.

Plate 4

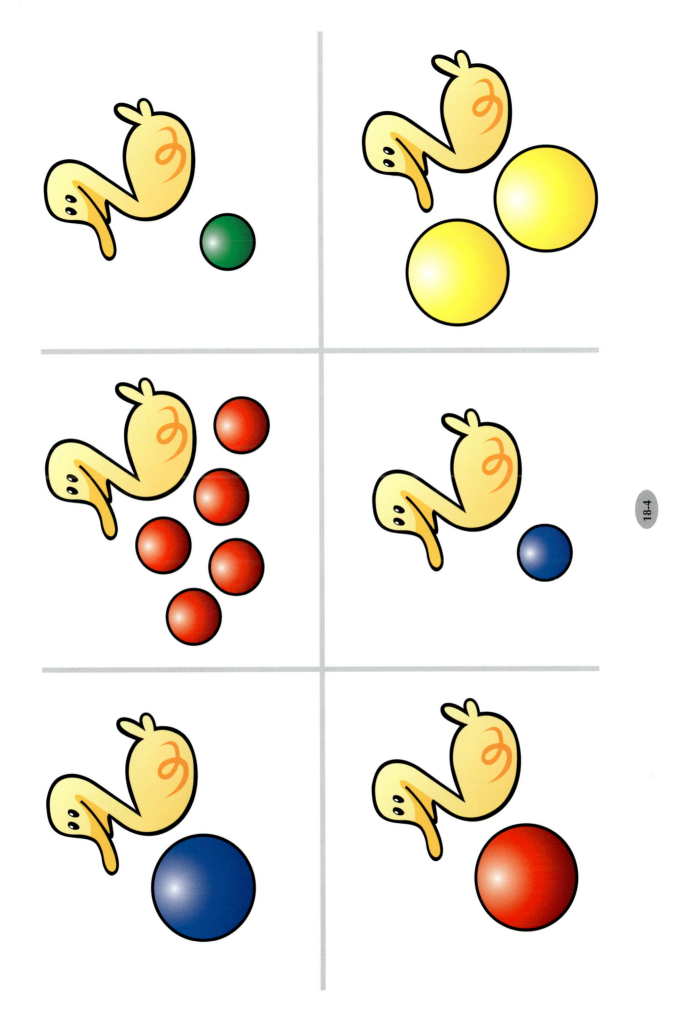

Level 1

Sublevel 18

noun + (size + color + singular/plural)

Example: Touch the bear with a big, green balloon.

1. Touch the bear with the little, yellow balloons.

2. Touch the bear with a big, red balloon.

3. Touch the bear with the little, green balloons.

4. Touch the bear with a big, green balloon.

5. Touch the bear with a little, blue balloon.

6. Touch the bear with the big, red balloons.

Plate 5

©2012 Super Duper® Publications

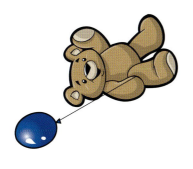
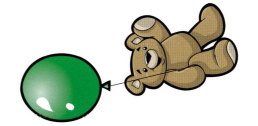
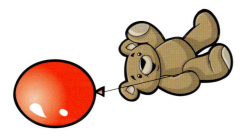
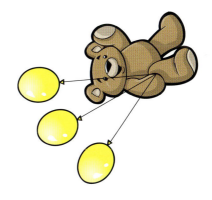

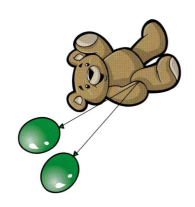
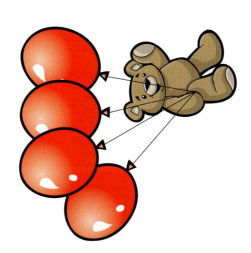

Level 1

Plate 6

Sublevel 18

noun + (size + color + singular/plural)

Example: Touch the dog with a big, green book.

1. Touch the dog with a big, blue book.

2. Touch the dog with the big, yellow books.

3. Touch the dog with the little, yellow books.

4. Touch the dog with a little, red book.

5. Touch the dog with a big, green book.

6. Touch the dog with the little, green books.

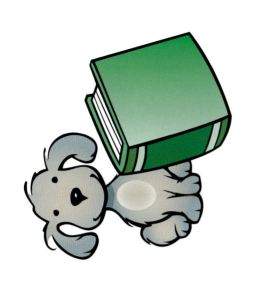
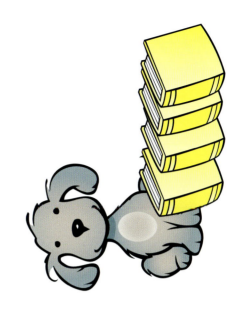
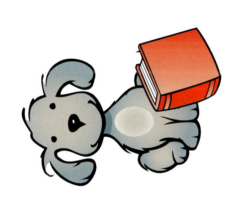
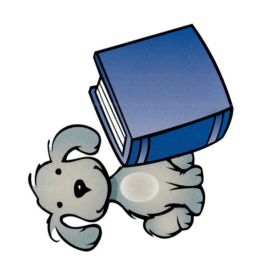
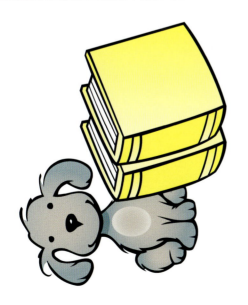
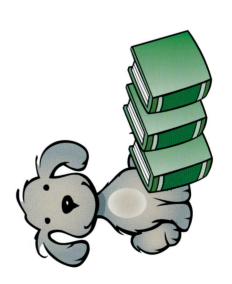

Level 1

Sublevel 18

noun + (size + color + singular/plural)

Example: Touch the sled with a big, green ring.

1. Touch the sled with the little, yellow rings.

2. Touch the sled with a big, blue ring.

3. Touch the sled with the little, red rings.

4. Touch the sled with the big, blue rings.

5. Touch the sled with a little, yellow ring.

6. Touch the sled with a big, green ring.

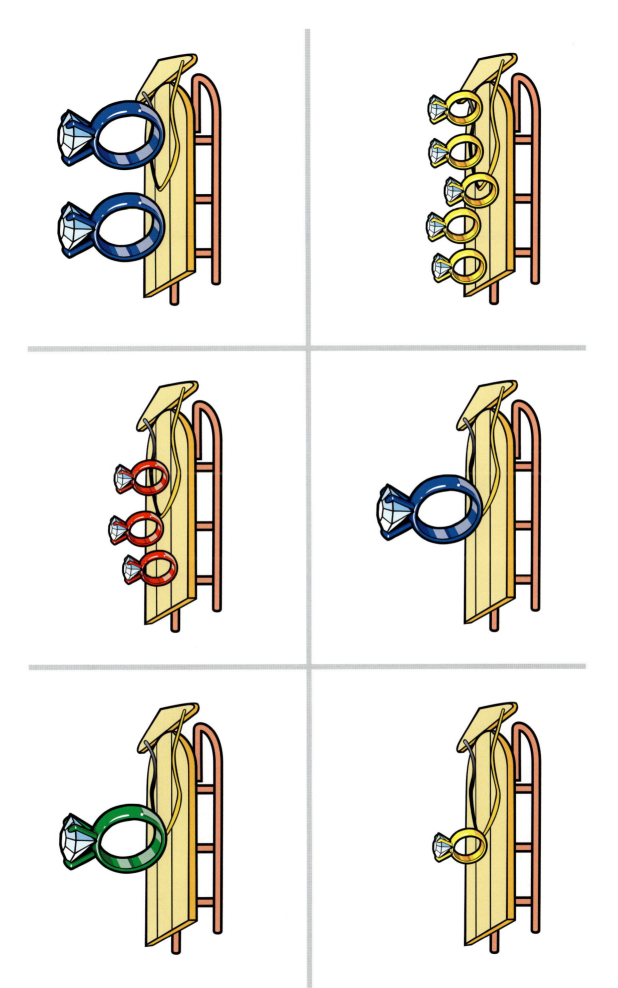

Level 1

Sublevel 19

noun + (preposition + noun)
Example: *Touch the mouse under a hat.*

1. Touch the cat under a hat.

2. Touch the mouse in a hat.

3. Touch the cat in a hat.

4. Touch the mouse on a hat.

5. Touch the cat on a hat.

6. Touch the mouse under a hat.

Plate 1

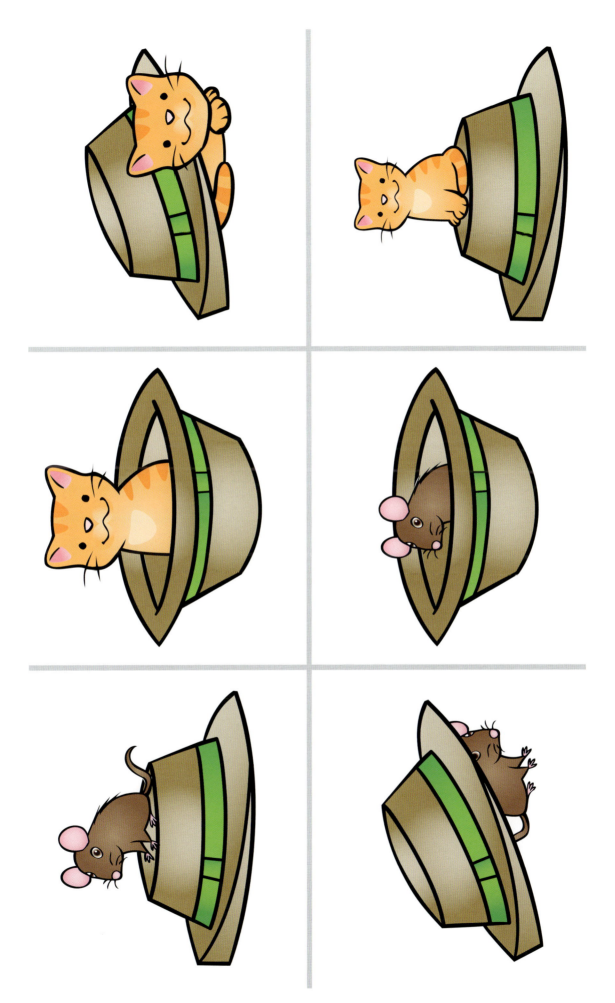

Level 1

Sublevel 19

noun + (preposition + noun)

Example: Touch the dog on a bowl.

1. Touch the dog under a bowl.
2. Touch the dog on a bowl.
3. Touch the bear in a bowl.
4. Touch the dog in a bowl.
5. Touch the bear on a bowl.
6. Touch the bear under a bowl.

Plate 2

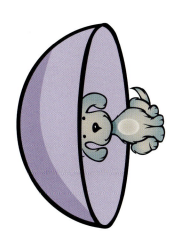
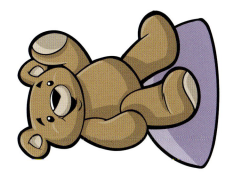
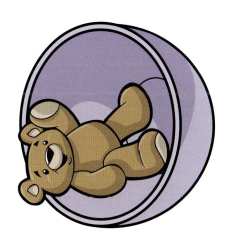
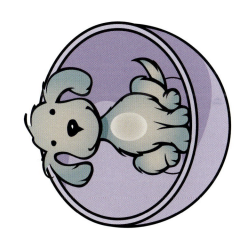
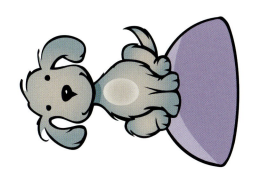
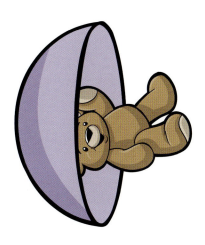

Level 1

Sublevel 19

noun + (preposition + noun)

Example: *Touch the duck on a cup.*

1. Touch the duck under a cup.

2. Touch the frog in a cup.

3. Touch the duck on a cup.

4. Touch the frog on a cup.

5. Touch the duck in a cup.

6. Touch the frog under a cup.

Plate 3

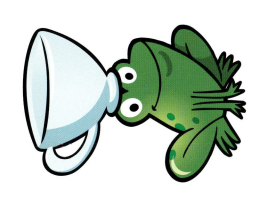
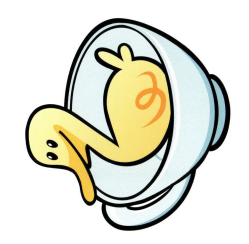
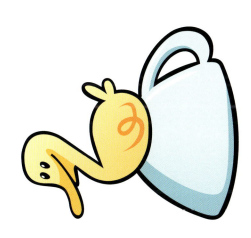
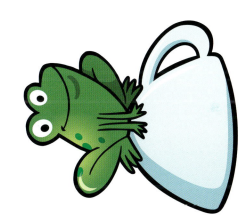

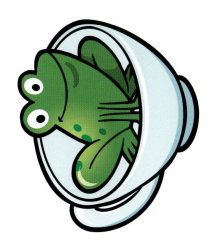
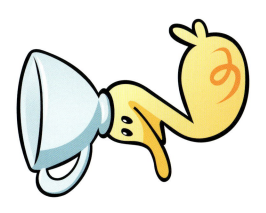

Level 1

Sublevel 19

noun + (preposition + noun)

Example: Touch the cat on a cup.

1. Touch the dog in a cup.
2. Touch the cat in a hat.
3. Touch the dog under a hat.
4. Touch the cat on a cup.
5. Touch the dog on a hat.
6. Touch the cat under a cup.

Plate 4

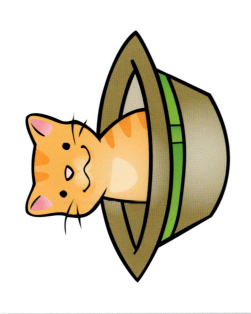
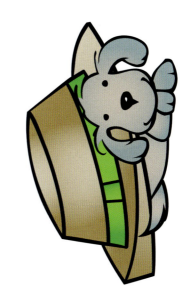
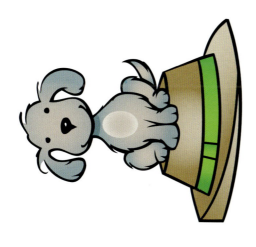
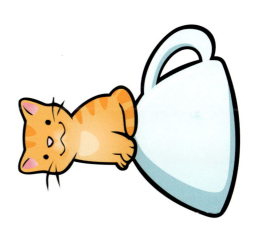
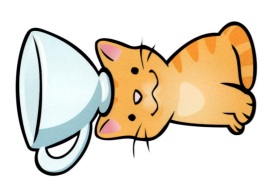
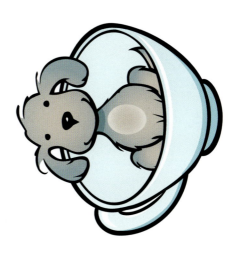

Level 1

Sublevel 19

noun + (preposition + noun)

Example: Touch the bear under a hat.

1. Touch the frog in a hat.
2. Touch the bear on a hat.
3. Touch the bear in a bowl.
4. Touch the frog under a bowl.
5. Touch the bear under a hat.
6. Touch the frog on a bowl.

Plate 5

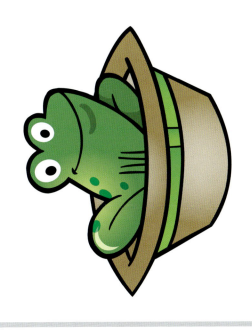
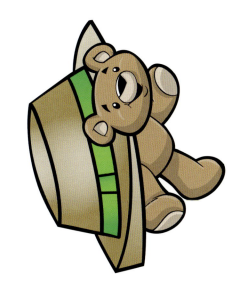
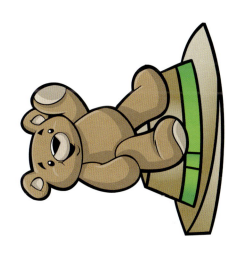
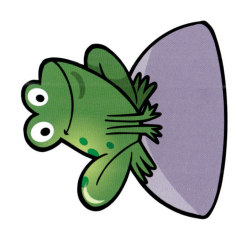
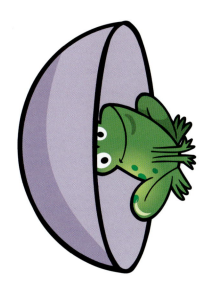
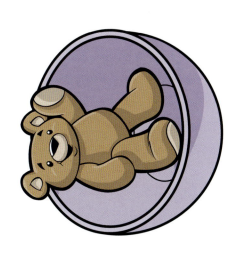

Level 1

Sublevel 19

noun + (preposition + noun)

Example: *Touch the mouse on a bowl.*

1. Touch the duck under a cup.
2. Touch the duck in a bowl.
3. Touch the mouse in a cup.
4. Touch the duck on a bowl.
5. Touch the mouse under a cup.
6. Touch the mouse on a bowl.

Plate 6

©2012 Super Duper® Publications

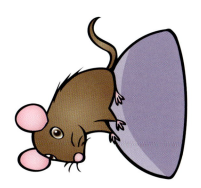
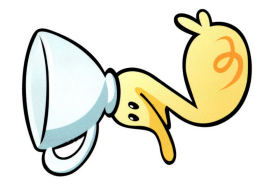
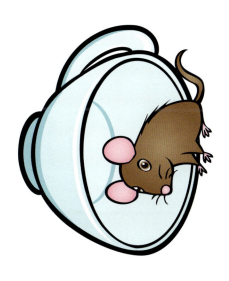
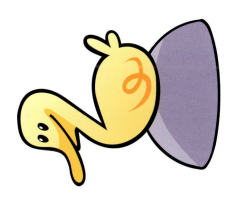
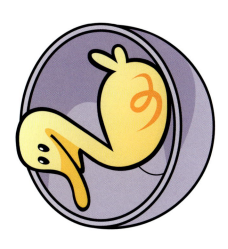
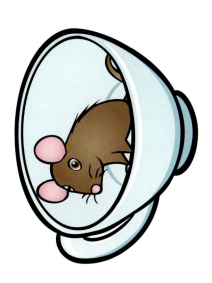

Level 1

Sublevel 20

singular/plural + (preposition + noun)

Example: Touch the rings that are on a cup.

1. Touch the rings that are in a cup.
2. Touch the ring that is in a cup.
3. Touch the ring that is under a cup.
4. Touch the rings that are on a cup.
5. Touch the ring that is on a cup.
6. Touch the rings that are under a cup.

Plate 1

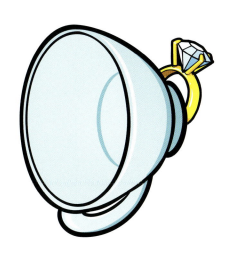
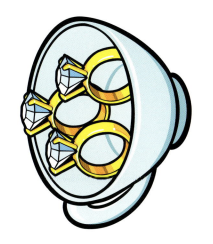
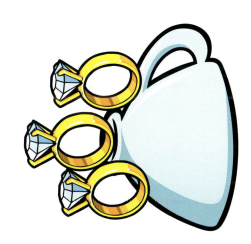
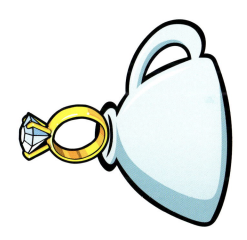
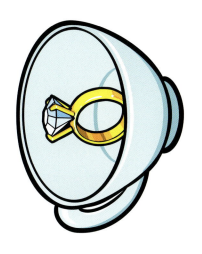
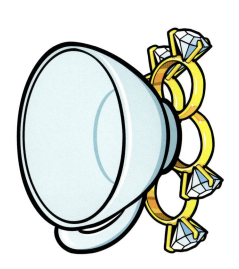

Level 1

Sublevel 20

singular/plural + (preposition + noun)

Example: Touch the buttons that are under a bowl.

1. Touch the button that is on a bowl.

2. Touch the buttons that are under a bowl.

3. Touch the button that is in a bowl.

4. Touch the buttons that are on a bowl.

5. Touch the buttons that are in a bowl.

6. Touch the button that is under a bowl.

Plate 2

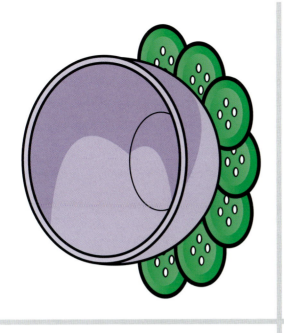
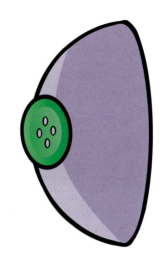
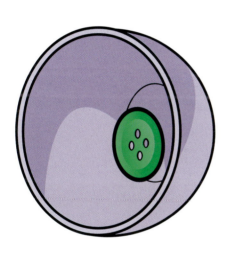
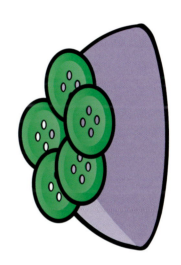
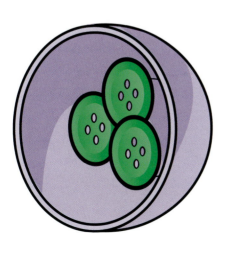
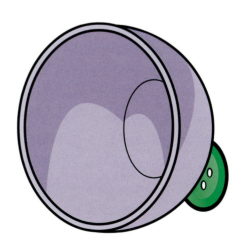

Level 1

Sublevel 20

singular/plural + (preposition + noun)

Example: Touch the books that are in a hat.

1. Touch the books that are under a hat.

2. Touch the book that is under a hat.

3. Touch the books that are in a hat.

4. Touch the book that is on a hat.

5. Touch the books that are on a hat.

6. Touch the book that is in a hat.

Plate 3

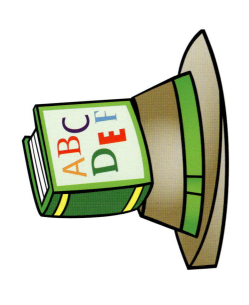
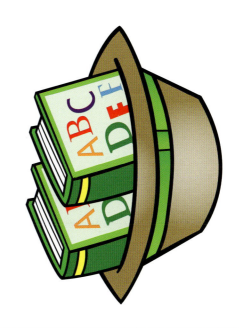
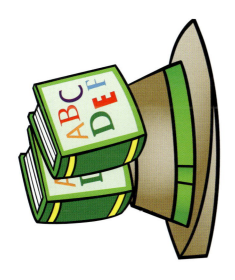
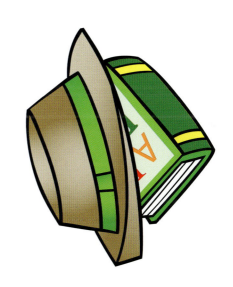

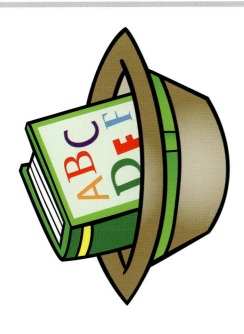
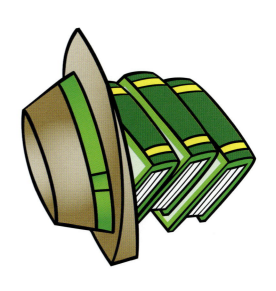

Level 1

Sublevel 20

singular/plural + (preposition + noun)

Example: Touch the beads that are in a bowl.

1. Touch the buttons that are on a bowl.

2. Touch the bead that is under a bowl.

3. Touch the button that is on a bowl.

4. Touch the beads that are in a bowl.

5. Touch the button that is under a bowl.

6. Touch the beads that are under a bowl.

Plate 4

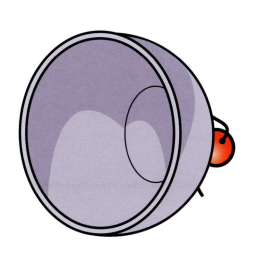
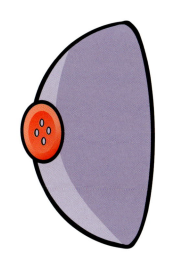
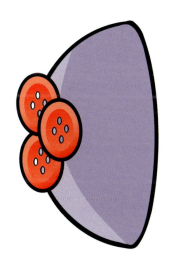
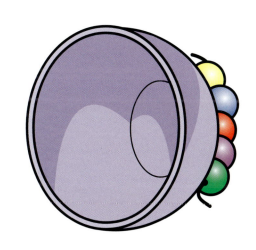
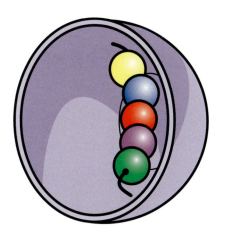
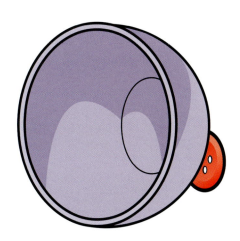
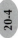

Level 1

Plate 5

Sublevel 20

singular/plural + (preposition + noun)

Example: Touch the books that are in a cup.

1. Touch the rings that are on a cup.

2. Touch the book that is on a cup.

3. Touch the ring that is under a cup.

4. Touch the book that is under a cup.

5. Touch the books that are in a cup.

6. Touch the rings that are under a cup.

©2012 Super Duper® Publications

236

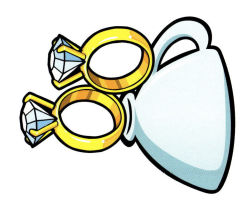
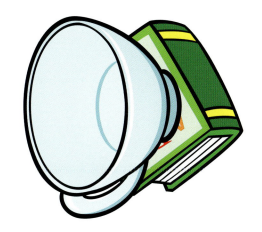
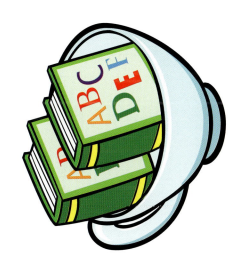
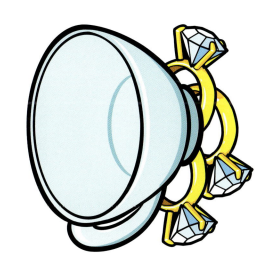
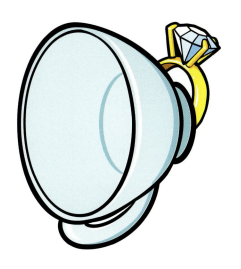
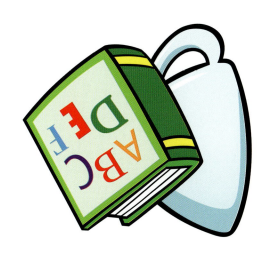

Level 1

Sublevel 20

singular/plural + (preposition + noun)

Example: Touch the socks that are under a hat.

1. Touch the mittens that are in a hat.
2. Touch the socks that are on a hat.
3. Touch the mitten that is in a hat.
4. Touch the sock that is under a hat.
5. Touch the mittens that are on a hat.
6. Touch the socks that are under a hat.

Plate 6

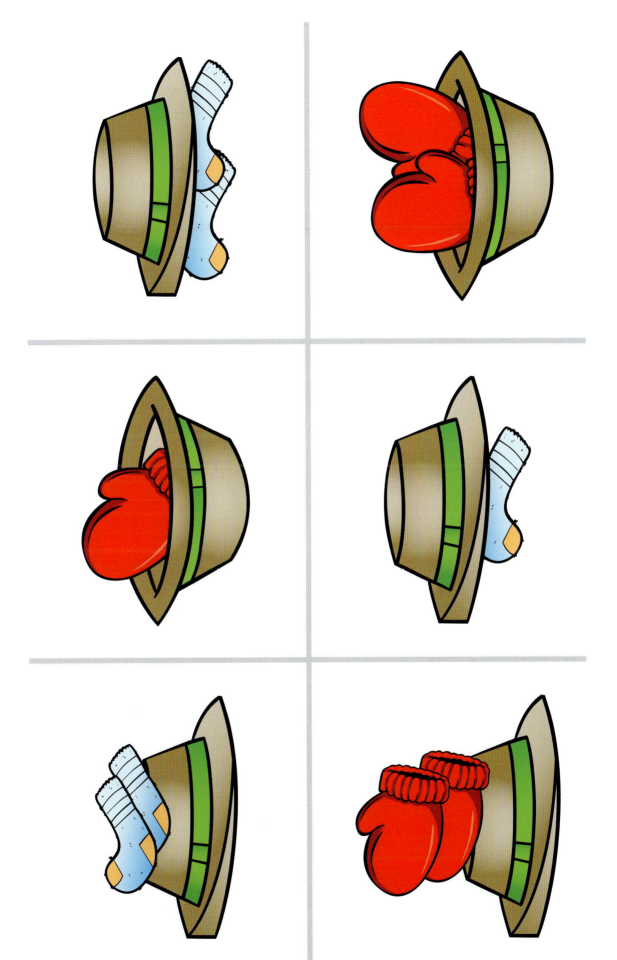

Level 1

Sublevel 21

(size + noun) + (preposition + noun)

Example: Touch the small ball in a cup.

1. Touch the big ball in a cup.
2. Touch the small ball on a cup.
3. Touch the big ball under a cup.
4. Touch the small ball under a cup.
5. Touch the big ball on a cup.
6. Touch the small ball in a cup.

Plate 1

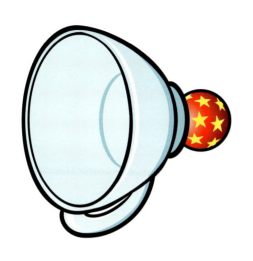
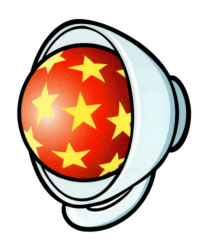
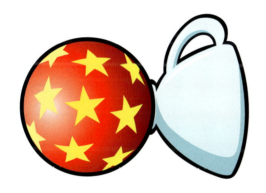
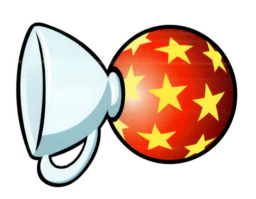
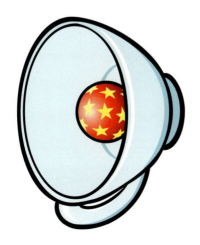
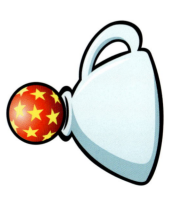
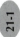

Level 1

Sublevel 21

(size + noun) + (preposition + noun)

Example: Touch the big mitten in a bowl.

1. Touch the small mitten in a bowl.
2. Touch the small mitten under a bowl.
3. Touch the big mitten under a bowl.
4. Touch the small mitten on a bowl.
5. Touch the big mitten in a bowl.
6. Touch the big mitten on a bowl.

Plate 2

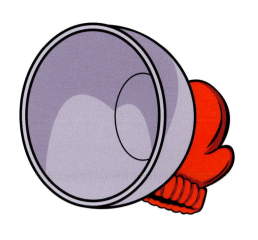
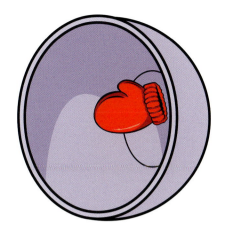
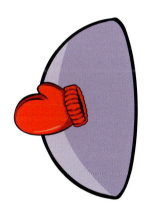
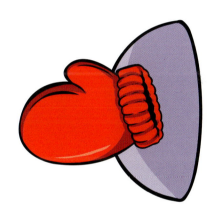
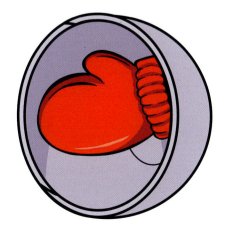
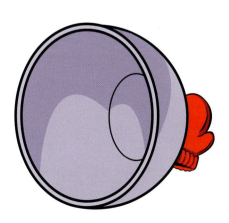

Level 1

Sublevel 21

(size + noun) + (preposition + noun)

Example: Touch the little duck on a hat.

1. Touch the little duck under a hat.
2. Touch the big duck on a hat.
3. Touch the little duck in a hat.
4. Touch the big duck in a hat.
5. Touch the little duck on a hat.
6. Touch the big duck under a hat.

Plate 3

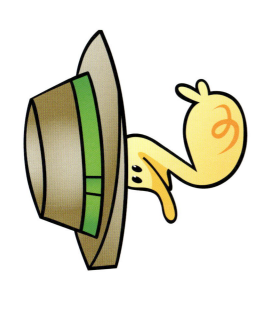
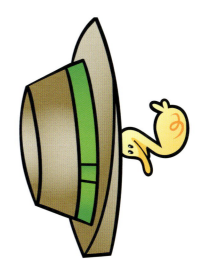
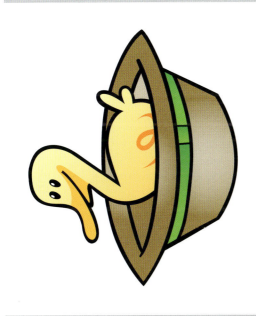
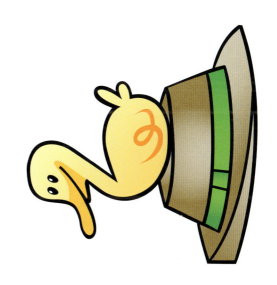

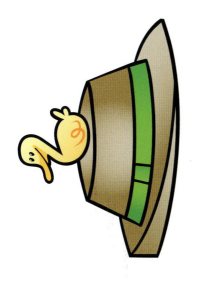
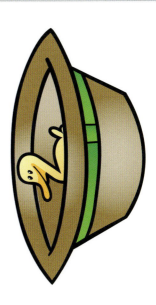

Level 1

Sublevel 21

(size + noun) + (preposition + noun)

Example: Touch the little shoe on a cup.

1. Touch the big sock on a cup.
2. Touch the little sock on a cup.
3. Touch the little sock under a cup.
4. Touch the big sock in a cup.
5. Touch the little sock in a cup.
6. Touch the big sock under a cup.

Plate 4

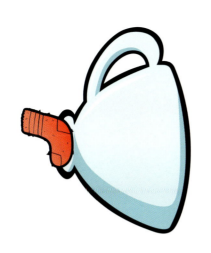
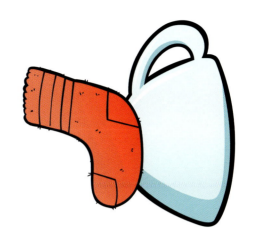
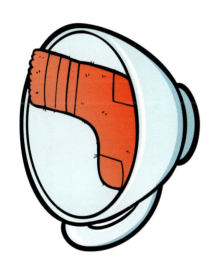
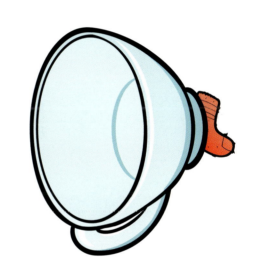
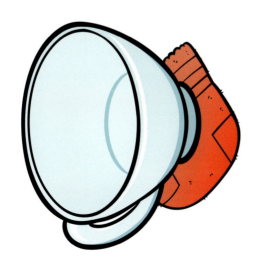
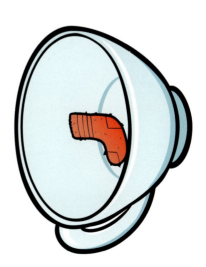

Level 1

Plate 5

Sublevel 21

(size + noun) + (preposition + noun)

Example: *Touch the big shoe on a bowl.*

1. Touch the big shoe under a bowl.
2. Touch the little shoe in a bowl.
3. Touch the big shoe on a bowl.
4. Touch the big shoe in a bowl.
5. Touch the little shoe on a bowl.
6. Touch the little shoe under a bowl.

©2012 Super Duper® Publications

248

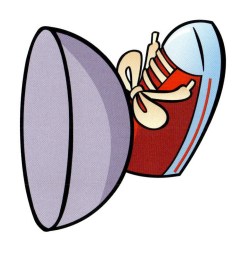
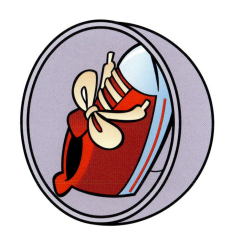
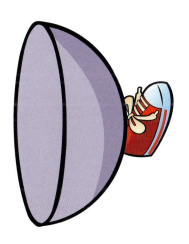
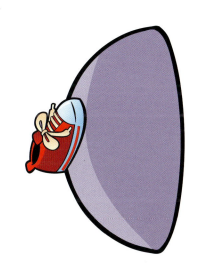
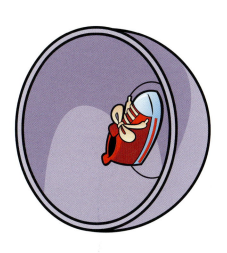
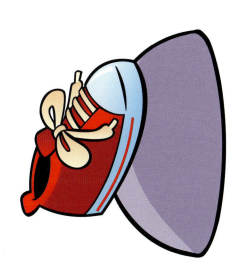

21-5

Level 1

Sublevel 21

(size + noun) + (preposition + noun)

Example: *Touch the little bear under a hat.*

1. Touch the little bear under a hat.

2. Touch the big bear in a hat.

3. Touch the little bear in a hat.

4. Touch the big bear under a hat.

5. Touch the little bear on a hat.

6. Touch the big bear on a hat.

Plate 6

©2012 Super Duper® Publications

250

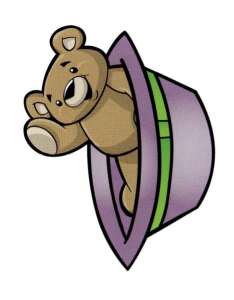
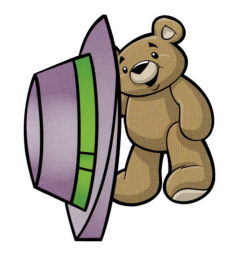
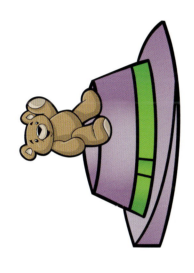
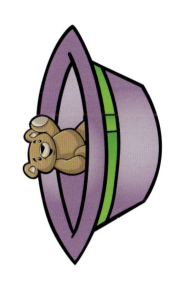
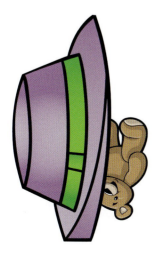
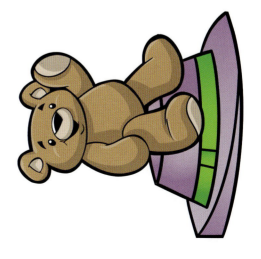

Level 1

Sublevel 22

(size + singular/plural) + (preposition + noun)

Example: *Touch the little cats on a hat.*

1. Touch the little cat in a hat.

2. Touch the big cat under a hat.

3. Touch the little cat on a hat.

4. Touch the big cats under a hat.

5. Touch the little cats on a hat.

6. Touch the big cats in a hat.

Plate 1

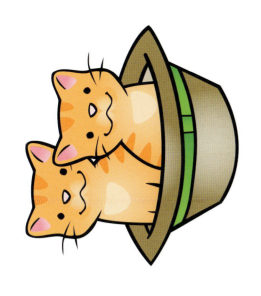
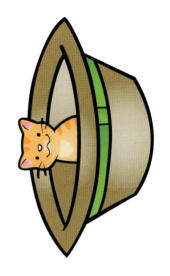
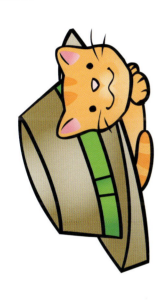
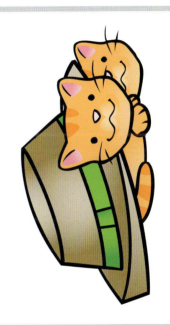
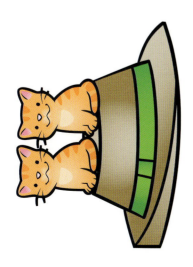
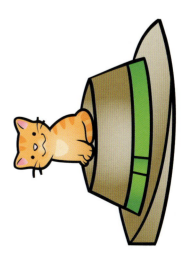

Level 1

Sublevel 22

(size + singular/plural) + (preposition + noun)

Example: Touch the small rings under a bowl.

1. Touch the small ring in a bowl.
2. Touch the small ring on a bowl.
3. Touch the big rings in a bowl.
4. Touch the small rings under a bowl.
5. Touch the big rings under a bowl.
6. Touch the big ring on a bowl.

Plate 2

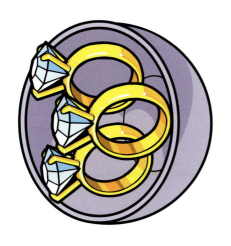
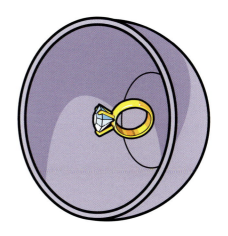
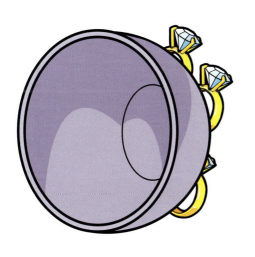
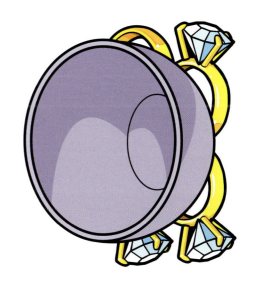
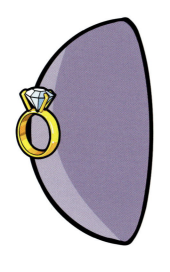
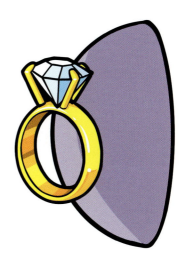

Level 1

Sublevel 22

(size + singular/plural) + (preposition + noun)

Example: Touch the big bead on a cup.

1. Touch the big bead under a cup.
2. Touch the little beads under a cup.
3. Touch the big bead on a cup.
4. Touch the big beads in a cup.
5. Touch the little bead on a cup.
6. Touch the little beads in a cup.

Plate 3

©2012 Super Duper® Publications

256

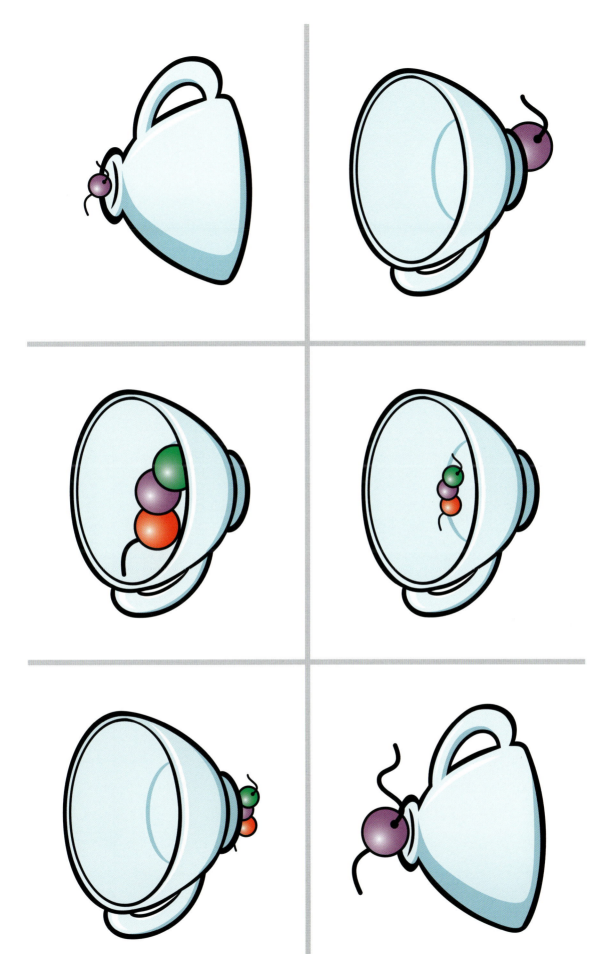

Level 1

Plate 4

Sublevel 22

(size + singular/plural) + (preposition + noun)

Example: Touch the little buttons in a bowl.

1. Touch the big button in a bowl.

2. Touch the big buttons under a bowl.

3. Touch the little buttons under a bowl.

4. Touch the little buttons in a bowl.

5. Touch the big button on a bowl.

6. Touch the little button on a bowl.

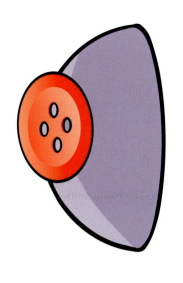
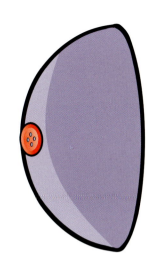
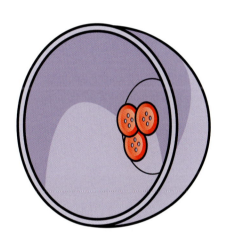
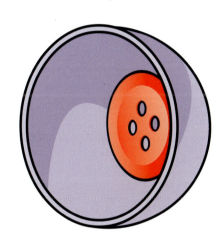

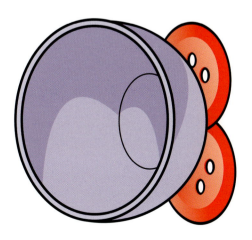
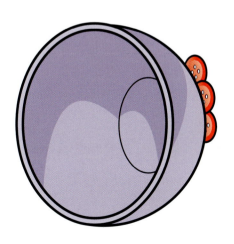

Level 1

Sublevel 22

(size + singular/plural) + (preposition + noun)

Example: Touch the little book on a cup.

1. Touch the big book in a cup.

2. Touch the little books in a cup.

3. Touch the big book on a cup.

4. Touch the big books under a cup.

5. Touch the little book on a cup.

6. Touch the little books under a cup.

©2012 Super Duper® Publications

Plate 5

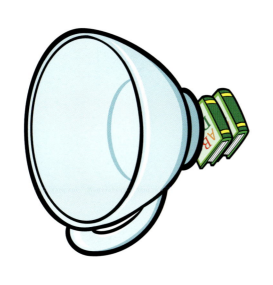
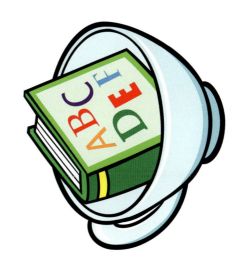
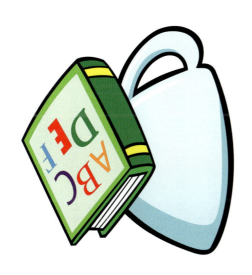
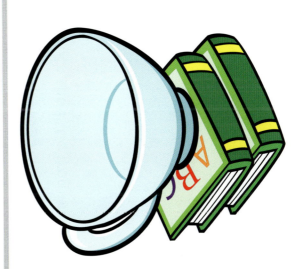
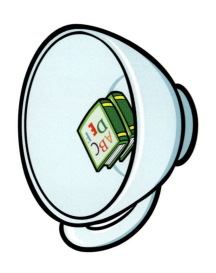
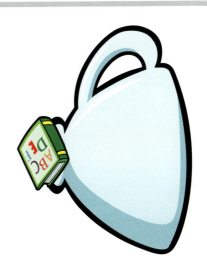

Level 1

Sublevel 22

(size + singular/plural) + (preposition + noun)

Example: Touch the little frog on a hat.

1. Touch the big frogs in a hat.

2. Touch the little frogs in a hat.

3. Touch the big frog on a hat.

4. Touch the little frog under a hat.

5. Touch the big frogs on a hat.

6. Touch the little frog on a hat.

Plate 6

©2012 Super Duper® Publications

262

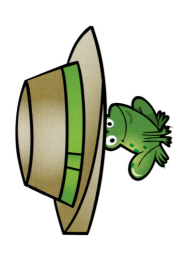
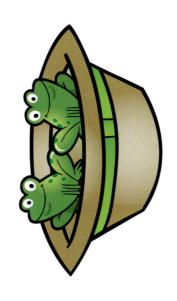
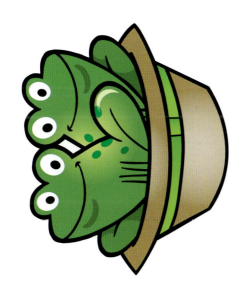
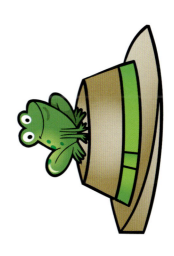
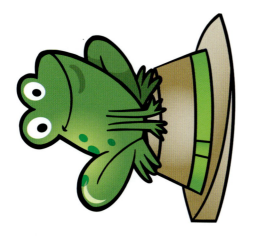
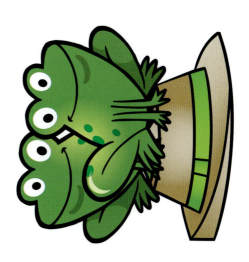

22-6

Level 1

Sublevel 23

(size + color + noun) + (preposition + noun)

Example: Touch the little, green ring in a cup.

1. Touch the big, red ring under a cup.

2. Touch the little, yellow ring under a cup.

3. Touch the big, red ring on a cup.

4. Touch the little, green ring in a cup.

5. Touch the big, green ring in a cup.

6. Touch the little, blue ring on a cup.

Plate 1

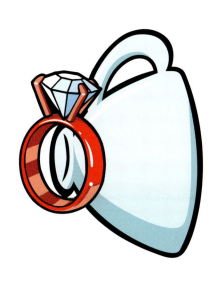
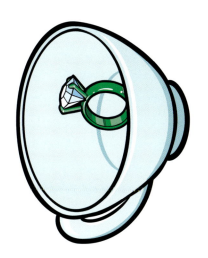
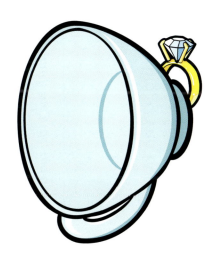
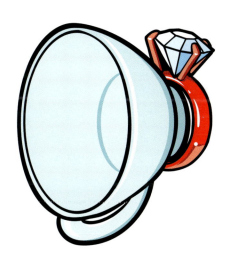
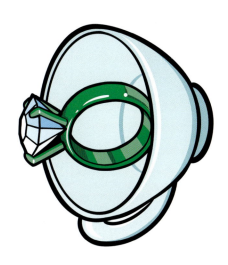
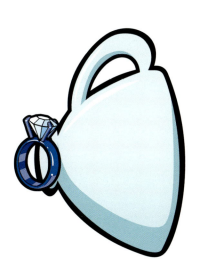

Level 1

Sublevel 23

(size + color + noun) + (preposition + noun)

Example: *Touch the little, red bead on a bowl.*

1. Touch the big, green bead on a bowl.

2. Touch the little, red bead on a bowl.

3. Touch the big, yellow bead under a bowl.

4. Touch the little, yellow bead under a bowl.

5. Touch the big, blue bead under a bowl.

6. Touch the little, blue bead in a bowl.

Plate 2

©2012 Super Duper® Publications

266

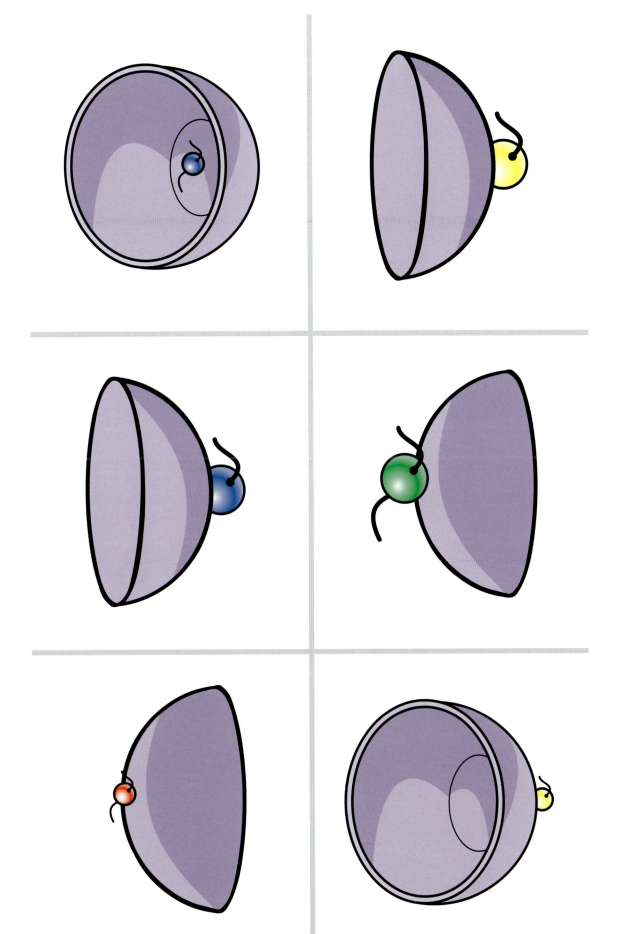

Level 1

Sublevel 23

(size + color + noun) + (preposition + noun)

Example: *Touch the big, green ball in a hat.*

1. Touch the big, blue ball on a hat.

2. Touch the little, yellow ball in a hat.

3. Touch the big, green ball in a hat.

4. Touch the big, red ball under a hat.

5. Touch the little, blue ball under a hat.

6. Touch the little, red ball on a hat.

Plate 3

©2012 Super Duper® Publications

268

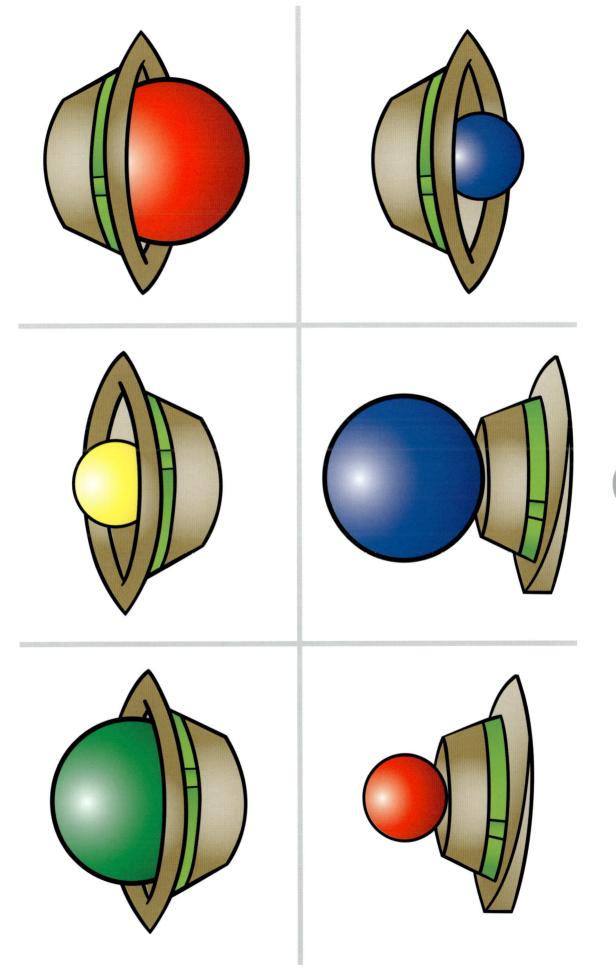

Level 1

Sublevel 23

(size + color + noun) + (preposition + noun)

Example: Touch the little, blue shoe in a bowl.

1. Touch the big, green shoe on a bowl.

2. Touch the big, red shoe under a bowl.

3. Touch the little, green shoe on a bowl.

4. Touch the little, blue shoe in a bowl.

5. Touch the big, yellow shoe in a bowl.

6. Touch the little, red shoe on a bowl.

Plate 4

©2012 Super Duper® Publications

270

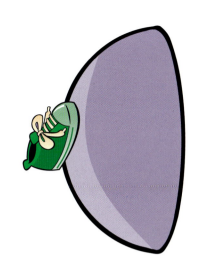
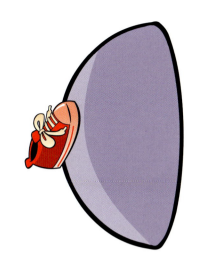
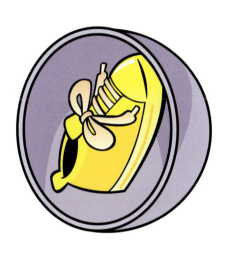
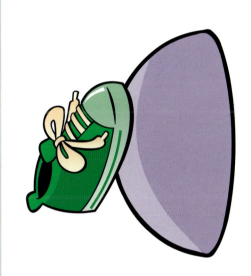
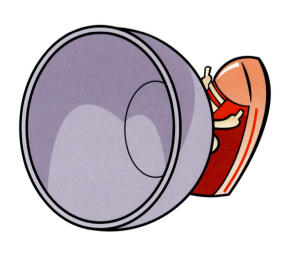
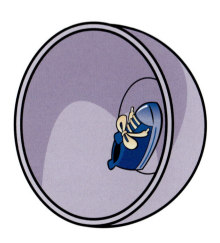

Level 1

Sublevel 23

(size + color + noun) + (preposition + noun)

Example: *Touch the little, blue button on a cup.*

1. Touch the little, green button on a cup.

2. Touch the big, blue button on a cup.

3. Touch the little, red button in a cup.

4. Touch the big, green button under a cup.

5. Touch the little, blue button on a cup.

6. Touch the big, yellow button in a cup.

Plate 5

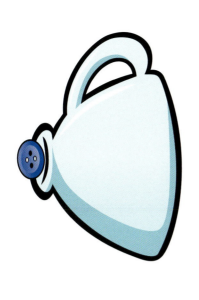
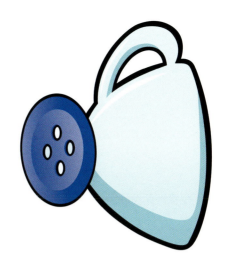
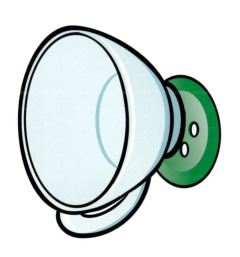
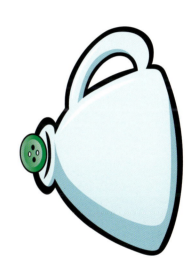
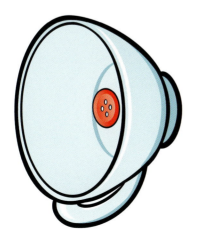
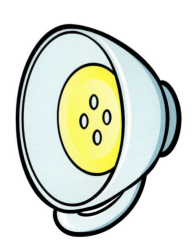

Level 1

Sublevel 23

(size + color + noun) + (preposition + noun)

Example: *Touch the big, blue sock on a hat.*

1. Touch the big, green sock under a hat.
2. Touch the little, blue sock in a hat.
3. Touch the little, red sock on a hat.
4. Touch the big, yellow sock in a hat.
5. Touch the little, yellow sock under a hat.
6. Touch the big, blue sock on a hat.

Plate 6

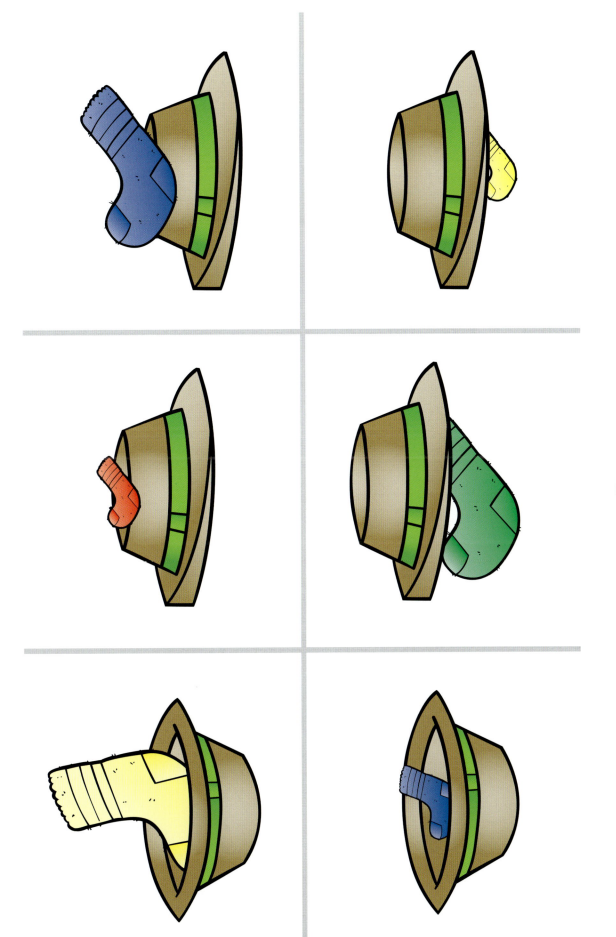

Level 1

Sublevel 24

(size + color + singular/plural) + (preposition + noun)

Example: Touch the big, red ring in a shoe.

1. Touch the little, red ring on a shoe.

2. Touch the little, green rings under a shoe.

3. Touch the big, red ring in a shoe.

4. Touch the big, yellow rings under a shoe.

Plate 1

©2012 Super Duper® Publications

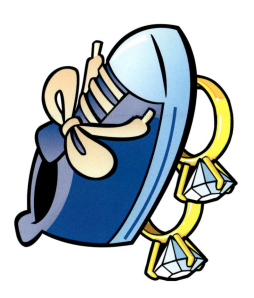
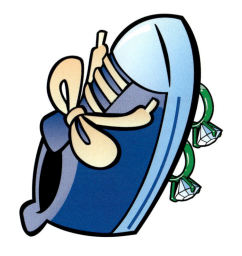
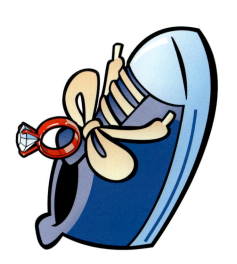
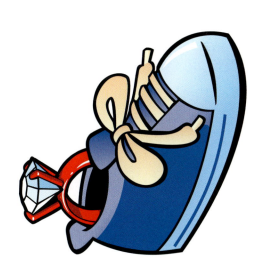

Level 1

Sublevel 24

(size + color + singular/plural) + (preposition + noun)

Example: Touch the big, red buttons under a cup.

1. Touch the little, blue button on a cup.

2. Touch the big, red buttons under a cup.

3. Touch the little, yellow buttons in a cup.

4. Touch the big, yellow button under a cup.

Plate 2

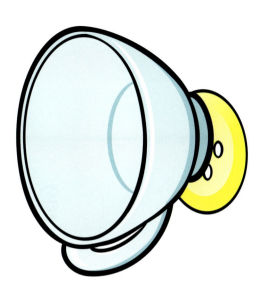
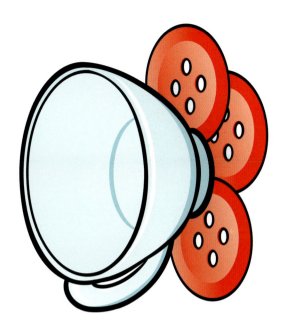
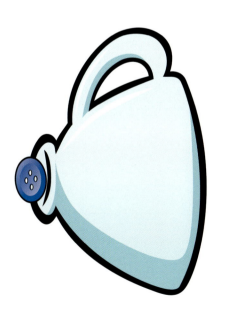
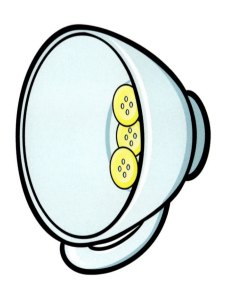

Level 1

Sublevel 24

(size + color + singular/plural) + (preposition + noun)

Example: Touch the little, green beads in a bowl.

1. Touch the big, blue beads under a bowl.

2. Touch the little, green beads in a bowl.

3. Touch the little, red bead on a bowl.

4. Touch the big, yellow bead on a bowl.

Plate 3

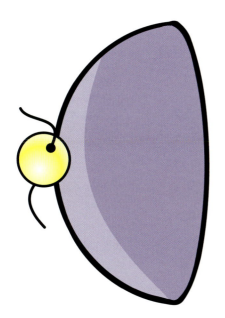
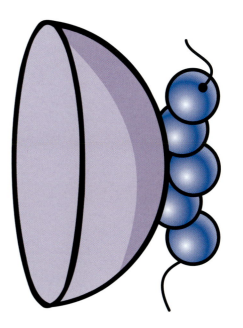
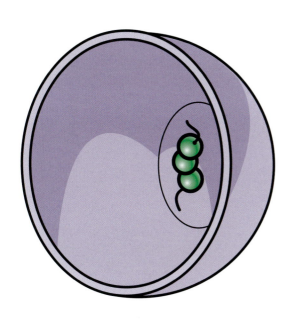
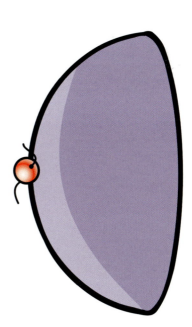

Level 1

Sublevel 24

(size + color + singular/plural) + (preposition + noun)

Example: *Touch the big, blue book in a cup.*

1. Touch the little, yellow book on a cup.

2. Touch the big, blue book in a cup.

3. Touch the little, green books under a cup.

4. Touch the big, yellow books in a cup.

Plate 4

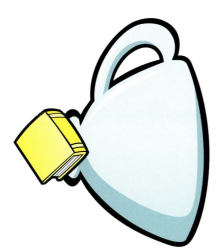
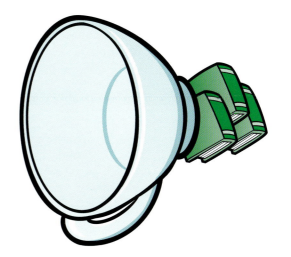
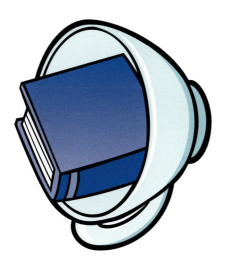
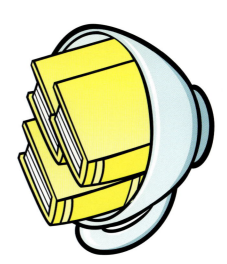

Level 1

Plate 5

Sublevel 24

(size + color + singular/plural) + (preposition + noun)

Example: Touch the big, blue mitten in a hat.

1. Touch the big, blue mitten in a hat.

2. Touch the little, yellow mitten under a hat.

3. Touch the big, blue mittens on a hat.

4. Touch the little, red mittens under a hat.

©2012 Super Duper® Publications

284

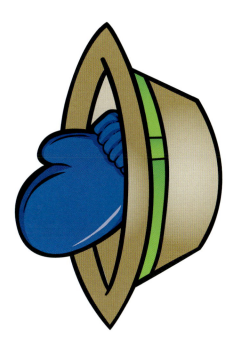
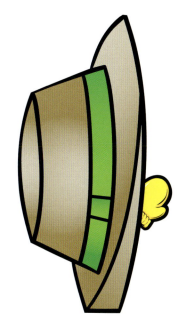
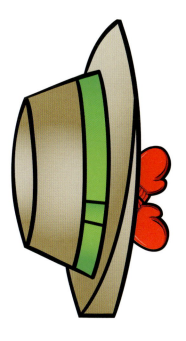
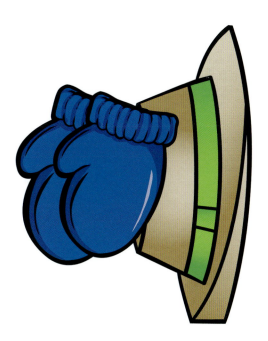
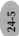

Level 1

Sublevel 24

(size + color + singular/plural) + (preposition + noun)

Example: Touch the little, red ball under a bowl.

1. Touch the little, green ball on a bowl.

2. Touch the big, red balls under a bowl.

3. Touch the big, green balls in a bowl.

4. Touch the little, red ball under a bowl.

Plate 6

©2012 Super Duper® Publications

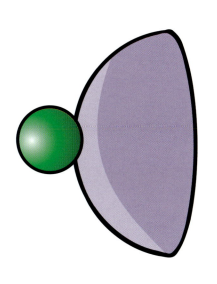
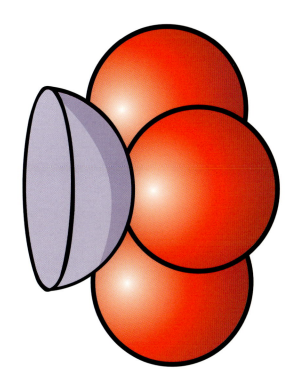
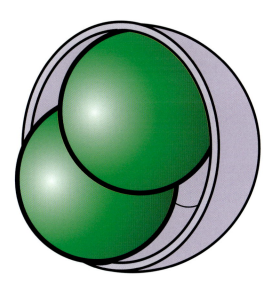
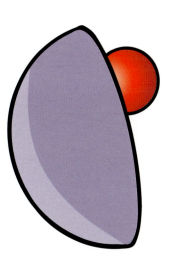

Level 1

Sublevel 25

quantity + size + singular/plural

Example: Touch one little airplane.

1. Touch one big airplane.

2. Touch some little airplanes.

3. Touch all the big airplanes.

4. Touch one little airplane.

5. Touch all the little airplanes.

6. Touch some big airplanes.

Plate 1

©2012 Super Duper® Publications

288

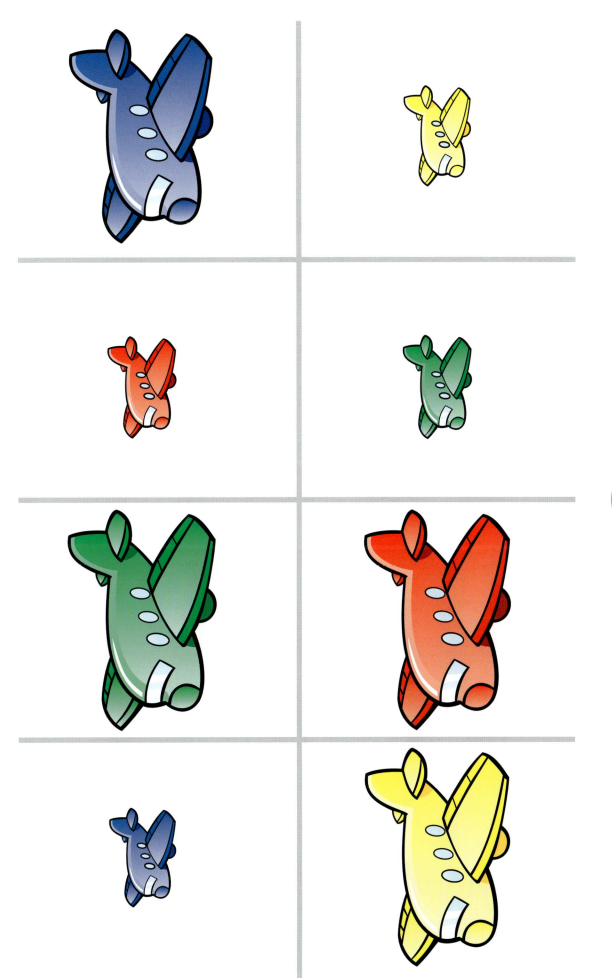

Level 1

Sublevel 25

quantity + size + singular/plural

Example: Touch some big balloons.

1. Touch some little balloons.

2. Touch one big balloon.

3. Touch all the little balloons.

4. Touch all the big balloons.

5. Touch some big balloons.

6. Touch one little balloon.

Plate 2

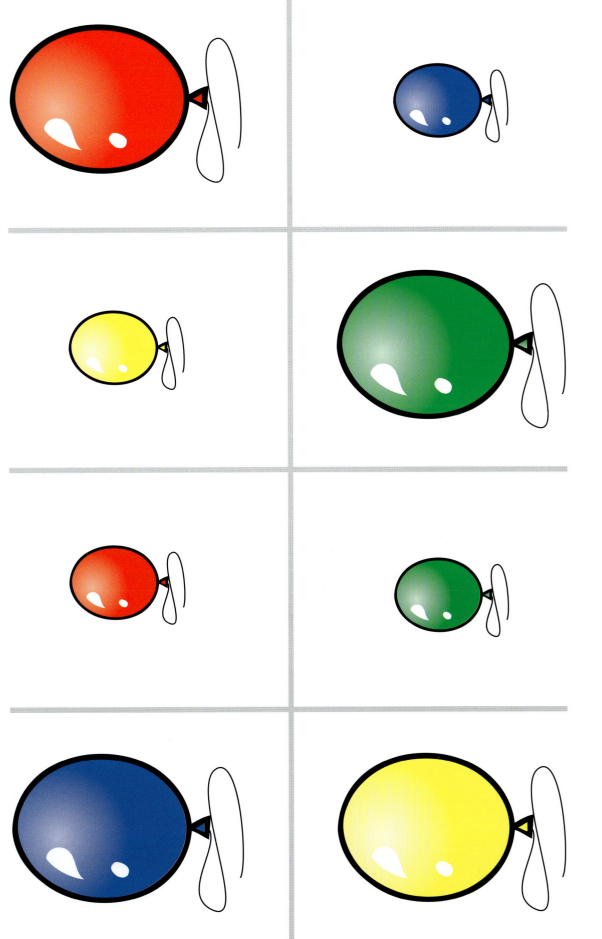

Level 1

Sublevel 25

quantity + size + singular/plural

Example: *Touch all the little dresses.*

1. Touch some big dresses.
2. Touch one little dress.
3. Touch one big dress.
4. Touch some big dresses.
5. Touch all the big dresses.
6. Touch all the little dresses.

Plate 3

©2012 Super Duper® Publications

292

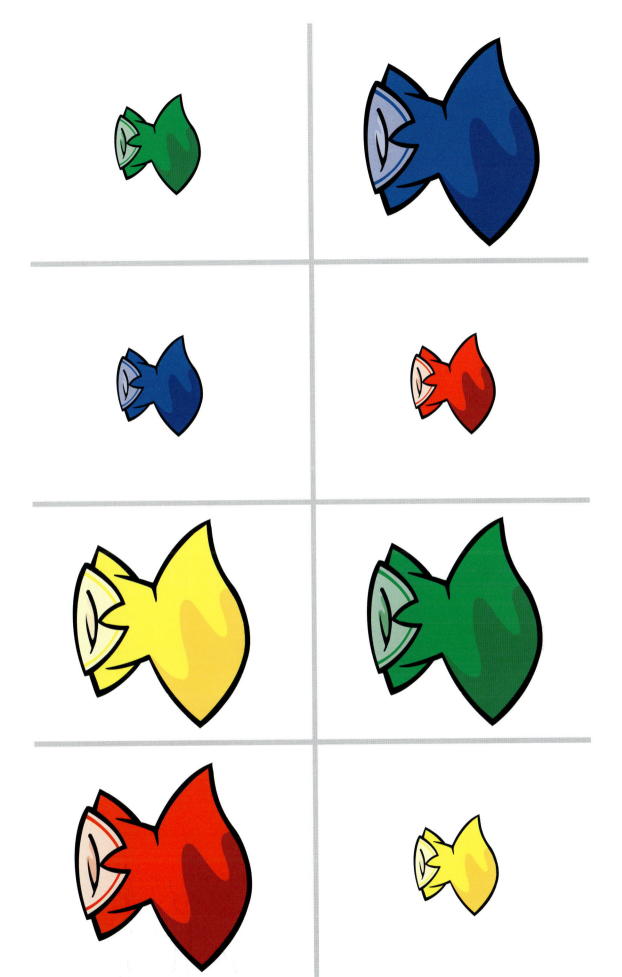

Level 1

Sublevel 26

noun + quantity + (color + noun)

Example: *Touch the mouse with the most red buttons.*

1. Touch the mouse with only blue buttons.
2. Touch the mouse with lots of red buttons.
3. Touch the mouse with a few green buttons.
4. Touch the mouse with the most green buttons.
5. Touch the mouse with no blue buttons.
6. Touch the mouse with a few yellow buttons.
7. Touch the mouse with lots of yellow buttons.
8. Touch the mouse with the most red buttons.

Plate 1

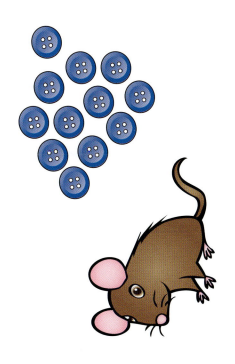
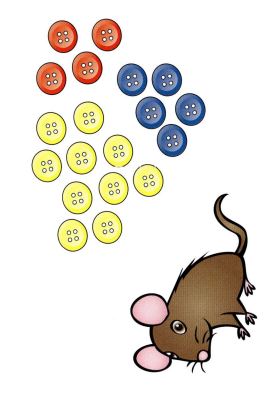
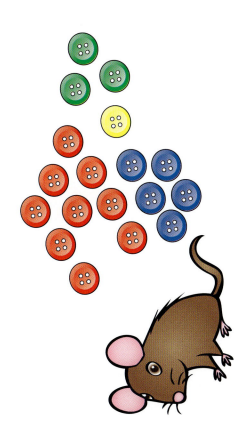
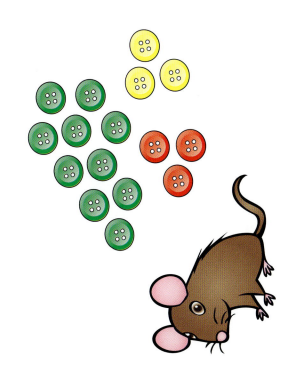
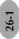

Level 1

Plate 2

Sublevel 26

noun + quantity + (color + noun)

Example: *Touch the hat with a few yellow balls.*

1. Touch the hat with the most yellow balls.

2. Touch the hat with no red balls.

3. Touch the hat with the fewest blue balls.

4. Touch the hat with the most blue balls.

5. Touch the hat with no yellow balls.

6. Touch the hat with lots of red balls.

7. Touch the hat with a few yellow balls.

8. Touch the hat with only green balls.

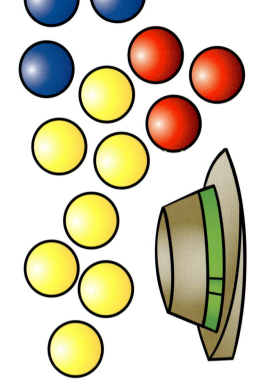
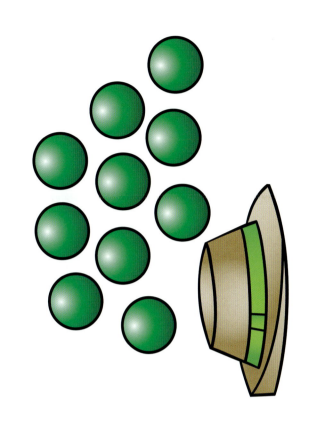
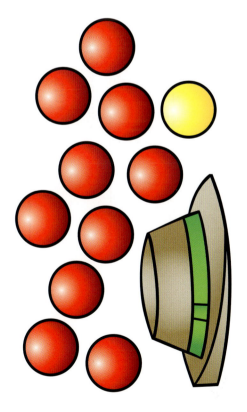
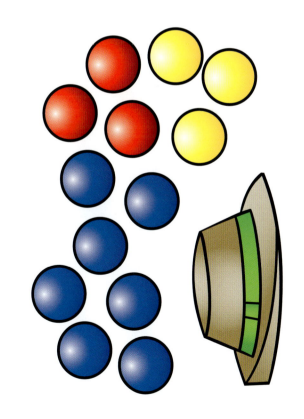

Level 1

Sublevel 26

noun + quantity + (color + noun)

Example: *Touch the cat with the fewest green rings.*

1. Touch the cat with the most yellow rings.

2. Touch the only cat with red rings.

3. Touch the cat with a few blue rings.

4. Touch the cat with the most blue rings.

5. Touch the cat with no blue rings.

6. Touch the cat with the fewest green rings.

7. Touch the cat with lots of green rings.

8. Touch the cat with no yellow rings.

©2012 Super Duper® Publications

Plate 3

298

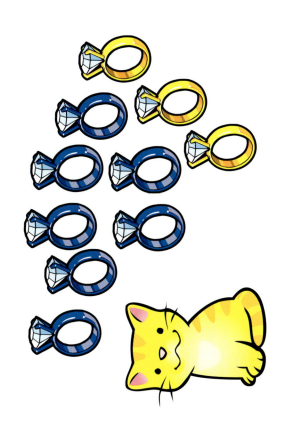
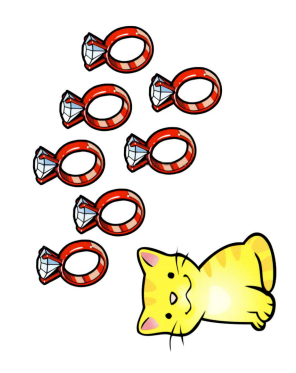
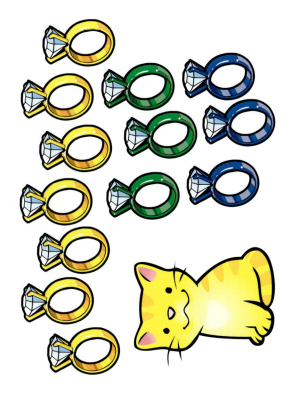
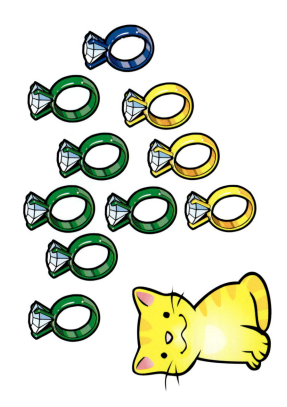

Level 1

Sublevel 26

noun + quantity + (color + noun)

Example: Touch the dress with a few green buttons.

1. Touch the only dress with red buttons.
2. Touch the dress with no blue buttons.
3. Touch the dress with the most yellow buttons.
4. Touch the dress with a few green buttons.
5. Touch the dress with only blue buttons.
6. Touch the dress with a few blue buttons.
7. Touch the dress with no yellow buttons.
8. Touch the dress with the most blue buttons.

Plate 4

©2012 Super Duper® Publications

300

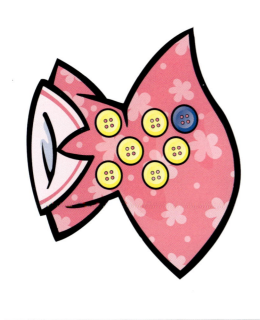
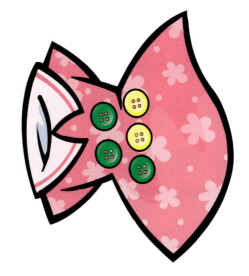
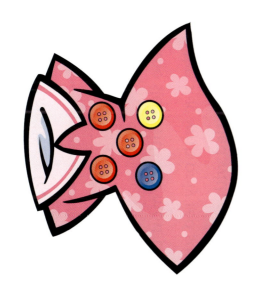
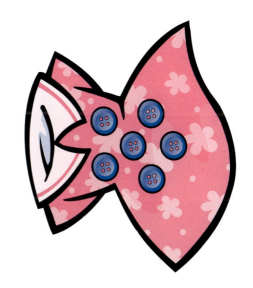
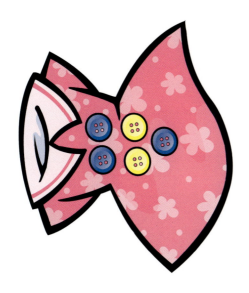
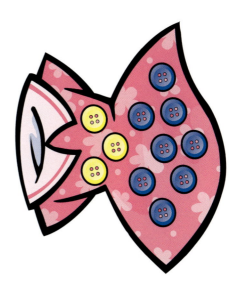
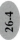

Level 1

Sublevel 26

noun + quantity + (color + noun)

Example: *Touch the only sled with green socks.*

1. Touch the sled with the most blue socks.
2. Touch the sled with only red socks.
3. Touch the only sled with green socks.
4. Touch the sled with no red socks.
5. Touch the sled with the most yellow socks.
6. Touch the sled with a few red socks.
7. Touch the sled with no blue socks.
8. Touch the sled with a few yellow socks.

Plate 5

©2012 Super Duper® Publications

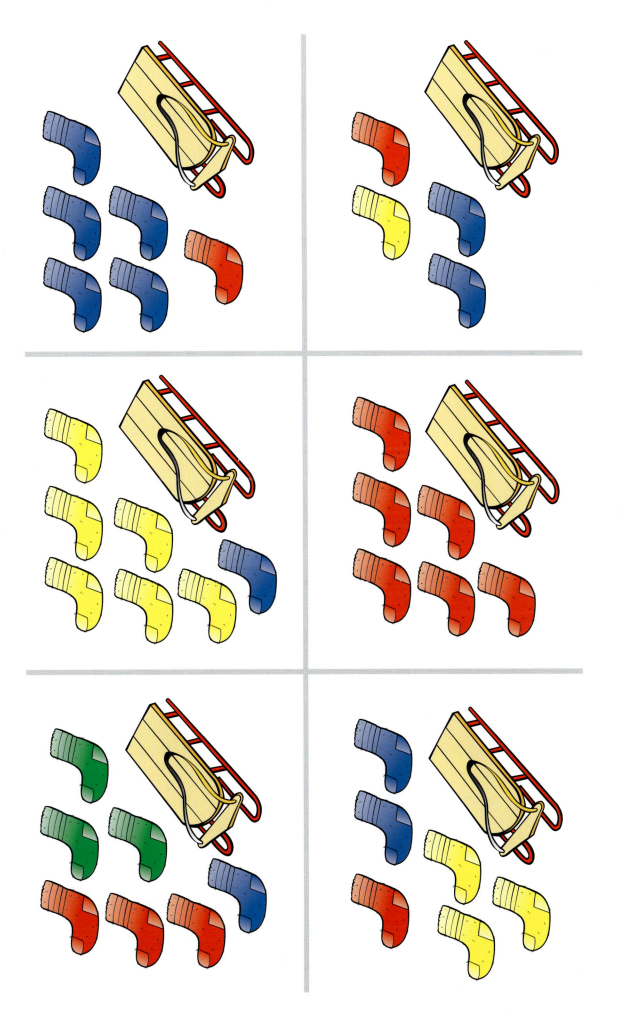

Level 1

Sublevel 26

noun + quantity + (color + noun)

Example: Touch the cup with a few green beads.

1. Touch the cup with a few yellow beads.

2. Touch the cup with only blue beads.

3. Touch the cup with a few green beads.

4. Touch the cup with the most yellow beads.

5. Touch the only cup with red beads.

6. Touch the cup with the fewest blue beads.

7. Touch the cup with no yellow beads.

8. Touch the cup with the most green beads.

Plate 6

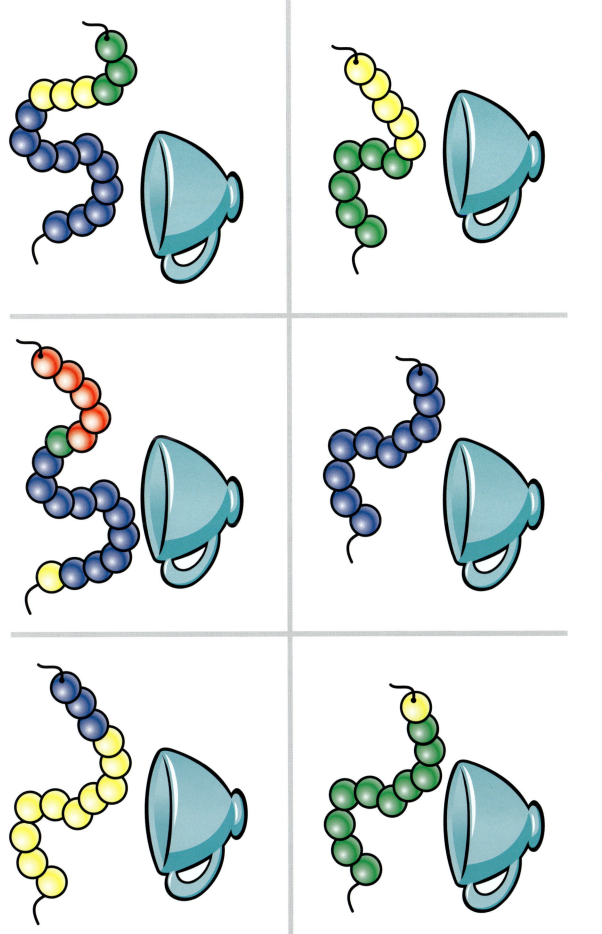

Level 1

Sublevel 27

noun + (quantity + size + noun)

Example: *Touch the dress with the fewest big buttons.*

1. Touch the dress with the most big buttons.
2. Touch the dress with the fewest little buttons.
3. Touch the dress with the most little buttons.
4. Touch the dress with the fewest big buttons.

Plate 1

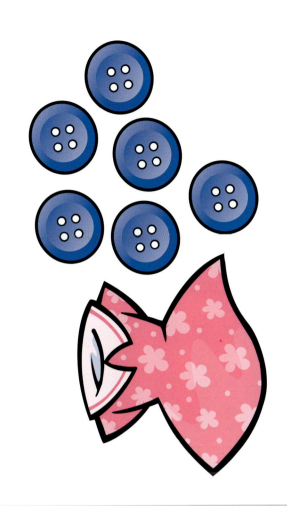
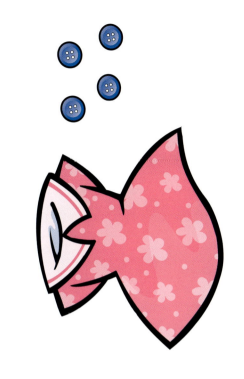
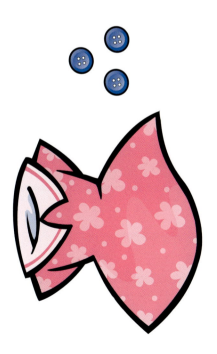
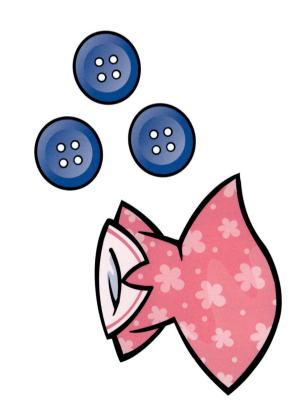

Level 1

Sublevel 27

noun + (quantity + size + noun)

Example: *Touch the sled with the most big cats.*

1. Touch the sled with the most little frogs.
2. Touch the sled with the fewest big cats.
3. Touch the sled with the most little cats.
4. Touch the sled with the fewest little frogs.
5. Touch the sled with the fewest little cats.
6. Touch the sled with the most big frogs.
7. Touch the sled with the most big cats.
8. Touch the sled with the fewest big frogs.

Plate 2

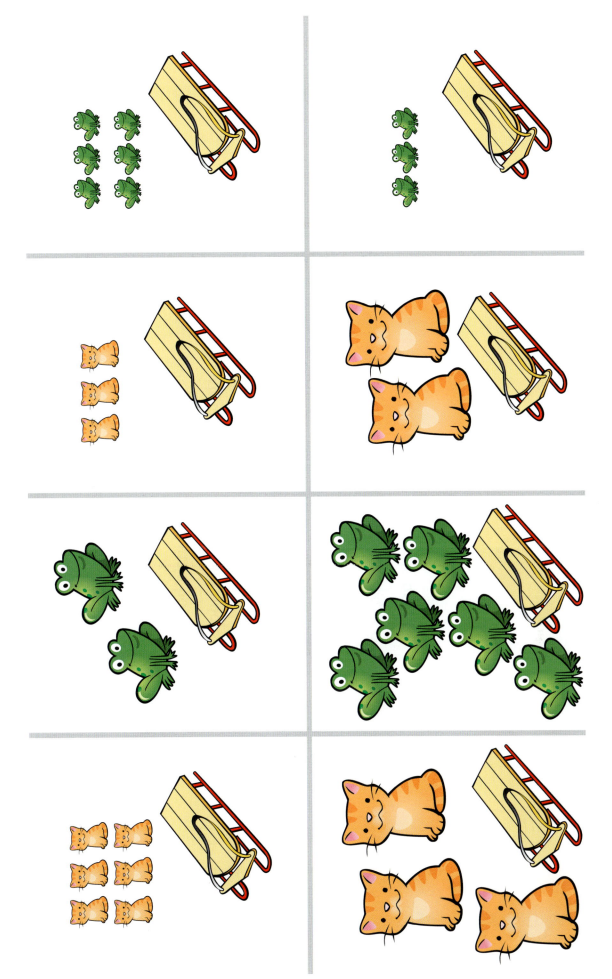

Level 1

Sublevel 28

noun + quantity + (size + singular/plural)

Example: Touch the bear with a few big books.

1. Touch the bear with no little books.

2. Touch all the bears with little books.

3. Touch the bear with only one big book.

4. Touch the bear with a few big books.

5. Touch the bear with only a little book.

6. Touch all the bears with big books.

7. Touch the bear with a few little books.

8. Touch some bears with little books.

Plate 1

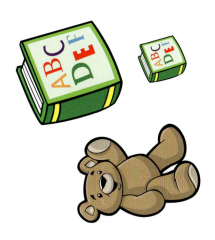
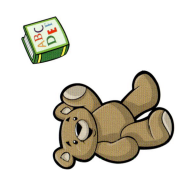
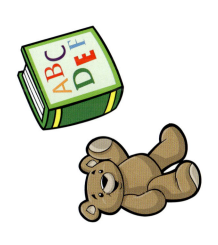
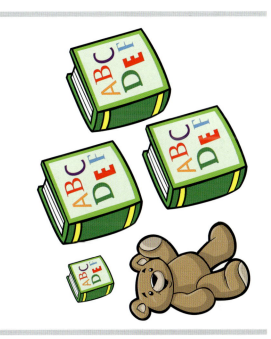
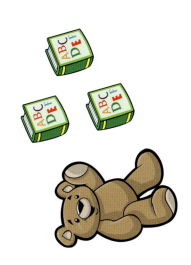
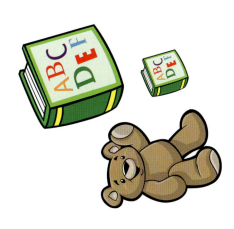

Level 1

Sublevel 28

noun + quantity + (size + singular/plural)

Example: Touch the dog with only big balloons.

1. Touch the dog with no little balloons.

2. Touch the dog with only little balloons.

3. Touch the dog with a few little balloons.

4. Touch the dog with only one big balloon.

5. Touch some dogs with big balloons.

6. Touch the dog with only big balloons.

7. Touch some dogs with little balloons.

8. Touch all the dogs with a big balloon.

Plate 2

©2012 Super Duper® Publications

312

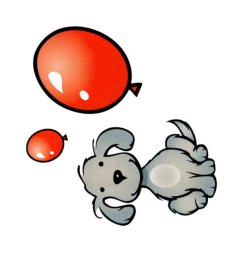
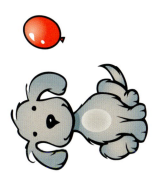
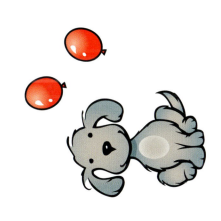
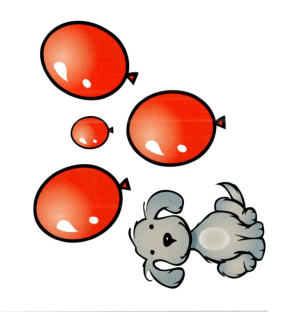

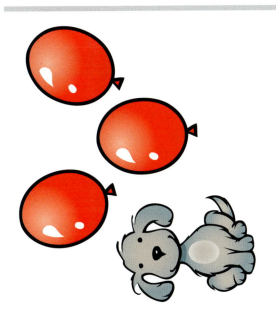
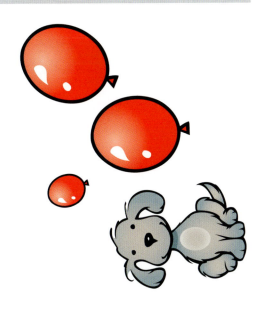

Level 1

Sublevel 28

noun + quantity + (size + singular/plural)

Example: Touch the hat with only big cats.

1. Touch the hat with only little cats.

2. Touch the hat with only one little cat.

3. Touch all the hats with big cats.

4. Touch the hats with no little cats.

5. Touch the hat with only one big cat.

6. Touch the hats with no big cats.

7. Touch the hat with only big cats.

8. Touch all the hats with little cats.

©2012 Super Duper® Publications

Plate 3

314

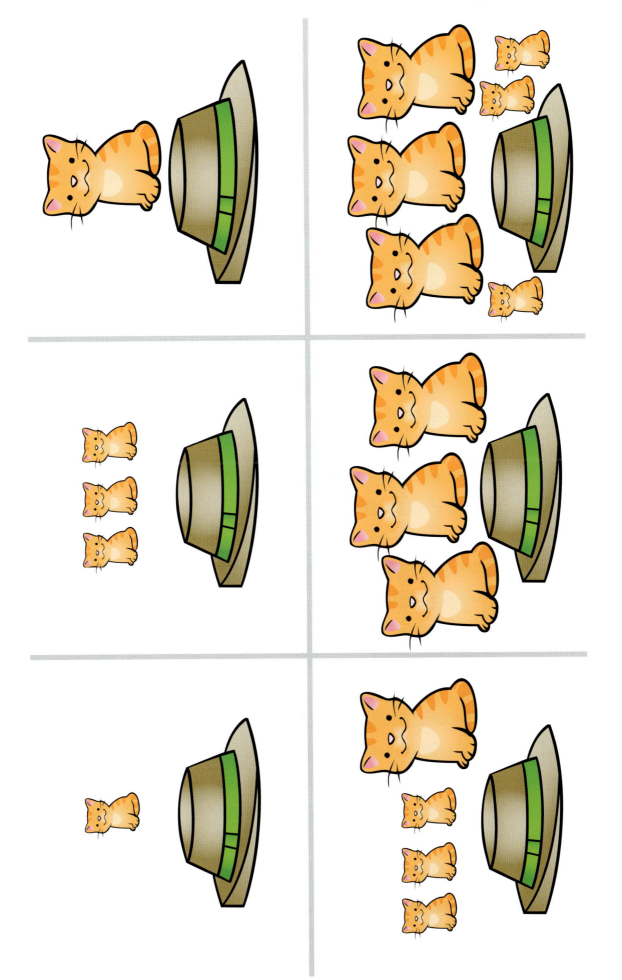

Level 1

Sublevel 28

noun + quantity + (size + singular/plural)

Example: Touch the cup with no big rings.

1. Touch all the cups with little rings.

2. Touch the cups with no little rings.

3. Touch the cup with only little rings.

4. Touch all the cups with big rings.

5. Touch some of the cups with little rings.

6. Touch the cup with only a big ring.

7. Touch the cups with a few little rings.

8. Touch the cups with a few big rings.

9. Touch the cup with no big rings.

Plate 4

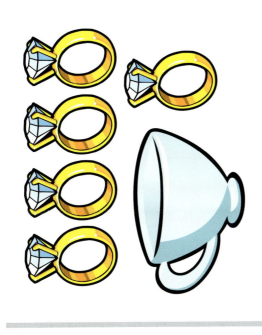
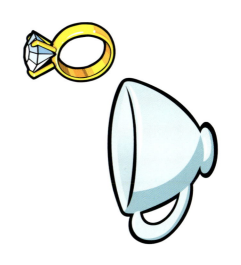
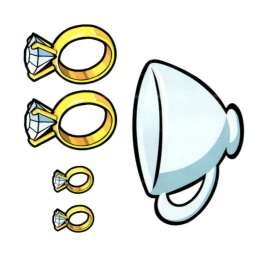
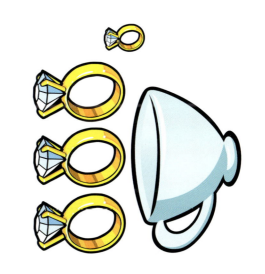
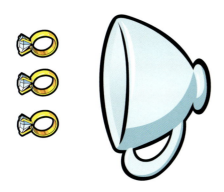
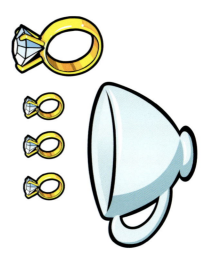
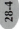

Level 1

Sublevel 29

(+/- **quantity** + **noun**) + **quantity** + (**size** + **color** + **singular/plural**)

Example: Touch the hat with only one, big, green ball.

1. Touch the hat with only big, red balls.

2. Touch all the hats with a few yellow balls.

3. Touch the hat with only little, blue balls.

4. Touch all the hats with little, yellow balls.

5. Touch some hats with no little, yellow balls.

6. Touch the hat with only one, big, green ball.

7. Touch all the hats with little, red balls.

8. Touch some hats with little, blue balls.

9. Touch the hat with the fewest little, blue balls.

Plate 1

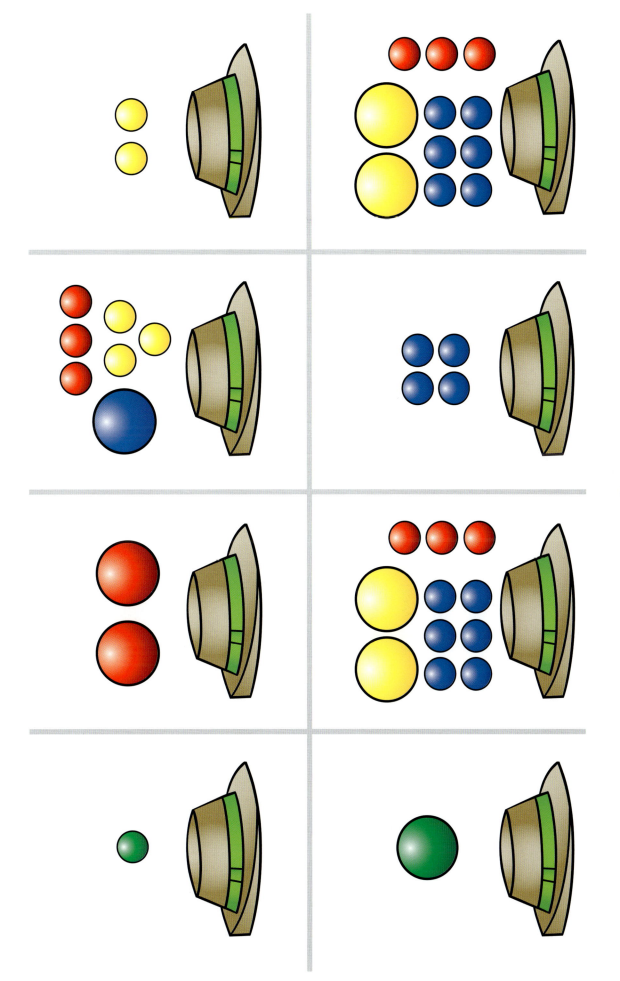

Level 1

Sublevel 29

(+/- quantity + noun) + quantity + (size + color + singular/plural)

Example: *Touch some cups with no little, yellow beads.*

1. Touch the cup with the most little, yellow beads.

2. Touch the only cup with big, green beads.

3. Touch the cup with the fewest little, blue beads.

4. Touch the cup with only big, red beads.

5. Touch the cups with a few little, green beads.

6. Touch all the cups with little, red beads.

7. Touch some cups with no little, yellow beads.

8. Touch the cups with a few big, yellow beads.

9. Touch the cup with the most little, red beads.

Plate 2

©2012 Super Duper® Publications

320

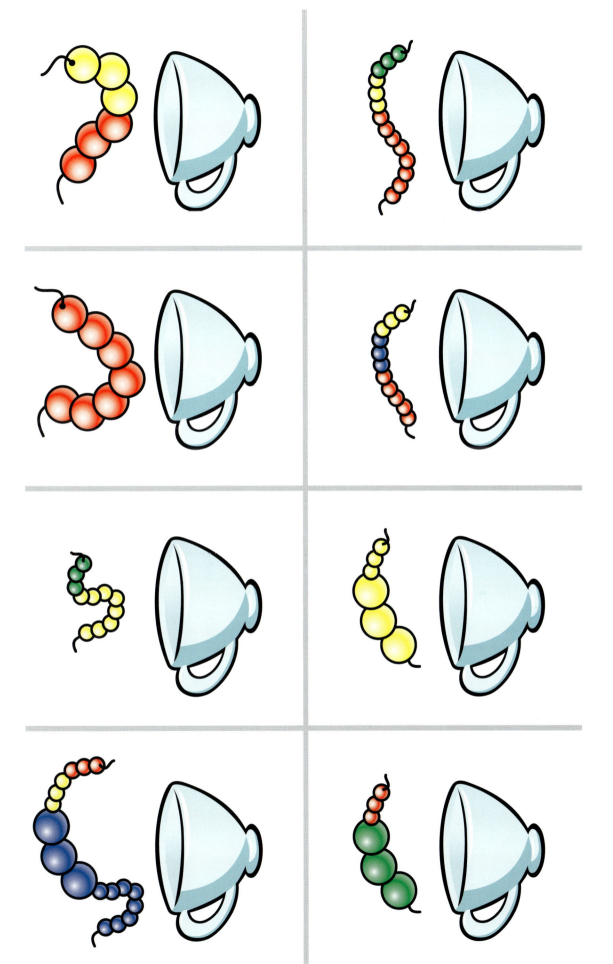

Level 1

Sublevel 29

(+/- quantity + noun) + quantity + (size + color + singular/plural)

Example: Touch the only dress with little, red buttons.

1. Touch the dress with the most big, blue buttons.

2. Touch the dress with no little, green buttons.

3. Touch all the dresses with big, yellow buttons.

4. Touch the dress with a few little, blue buttons.

5. Touch the dress with the most big, red buttons.

6. Touch some dresses with a few little, green buttons.

7. Touch the dress with only big, yellow buttons.

8. Touch the only dress with little, red buttons.

9. Touch all the dresses with big, blue buttons.

©2012 Super Duper® Publications

Plate 3

322

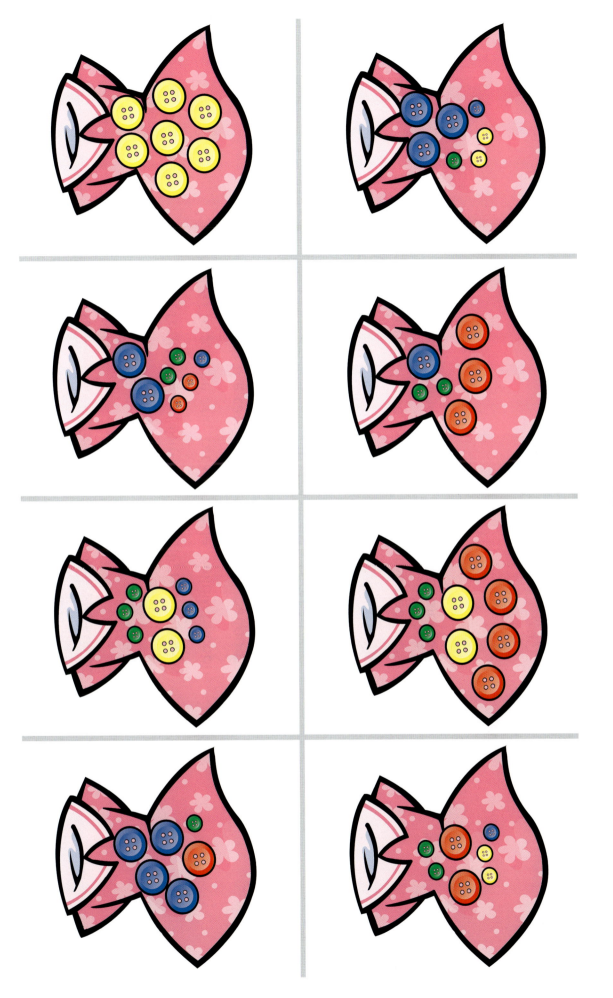

Level 1

Sublevel 29

(+/- quantity + noun) + quantity + (size + color + singular/plural)

Example: Touch all the cats with a few little, blue balloons.

1. Touch the cat with lots of little, red balloons.

2. Touch the only cat with little, yellow balloons.

3. Touch the cat with a few big, blue balloons.

4. Touch the only cat with one, big, red balloon.

5. Touch the cat with lots of little, green balloons.

6. Touch the cat with the fewest little, red balloons.

7. Touch the only cat with one, big, blue balloon.

8. Touch all the cats with little, green balloons.

9. Touch all the cats with a few little, blue balloons.

Plate 4

©2012 Super Duper® Publications

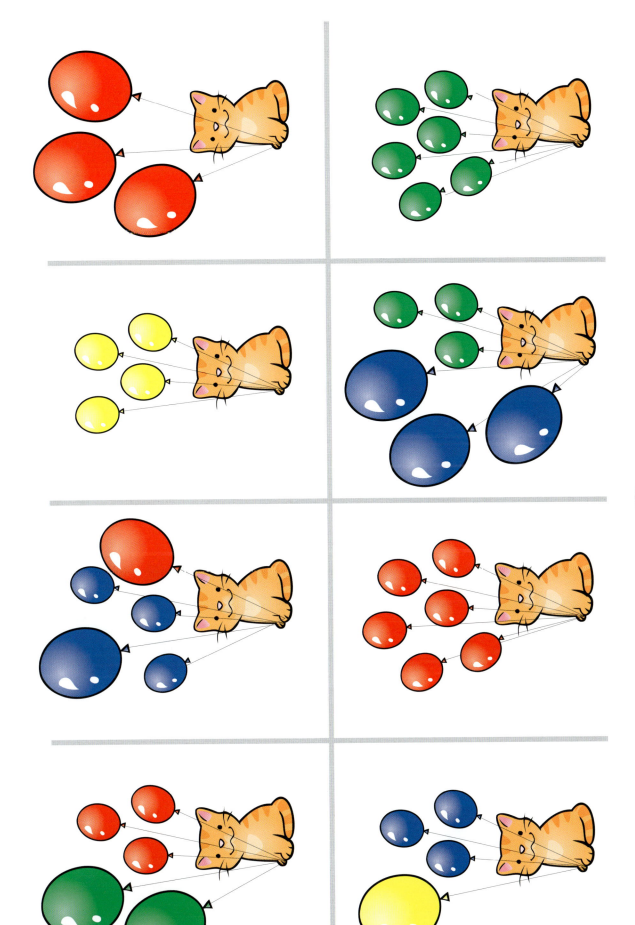

Level 1

Sublevel 30

(+/- quantity + singular/plural) +/- quantity + (size + color + noun) + (prep + pronoun)

Example: Touch the only cup with little, green beads in it.

1. Touch the cup with only little, red beads on it.
2. Touch the only cup with a few little, red beads on it.
3. Touch all the cups with no little, blue beads in them.
4. Touch the only cup with little, green beads in it.

Plate 1

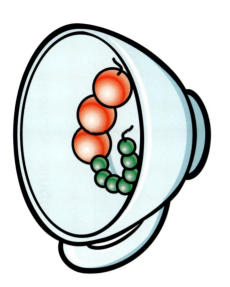
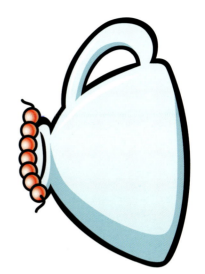
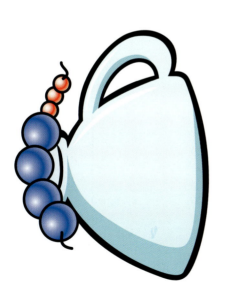
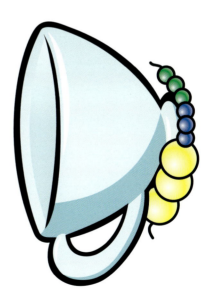
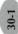

Level 1

Sublevel 30

(+/- quantity + singular/plural) +/- quantity + (size + color + noun) + (prep + pronoun)

Example: *Touch the cup with the fewest little, blue rings under it.*

1. Touch the cup with only big, green rings in it.

2. Touch the cup with the fewest little, blue rings under it.

3. Touch all the cups with big, green rings under them.

4. Touch the cup with a few little, green rings in it.

Plate 2

©2012 Super Duper® Publications

328

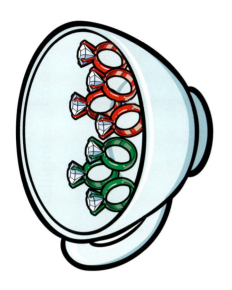
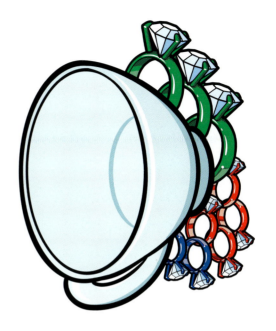
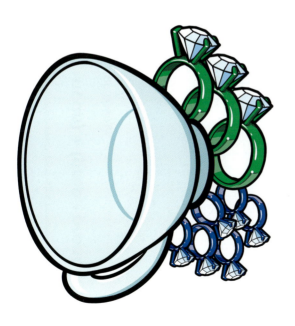
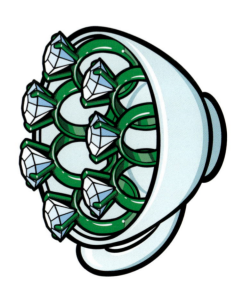

Level 1

Sublevel 30

(+/- quantity + singular/plural) +/- quantity + (size + color + noun) + (prep + pronoun)

Example: Touch all the hats with a few little, red cats on them.

1. Touch the hat with a few little, green cats in it.

2. Touch the hat with only big, yellow cats under it.

3. Touch all the hats with a few little, red cats under it.

4. Touch the hat with a few little, blue cats in it.

5. Touch the hat with the fewest big, yellow cats under it.

6. Touch the only hat with little, red cats under it.

Plate 3

©2012 Super Duper® Publications

330

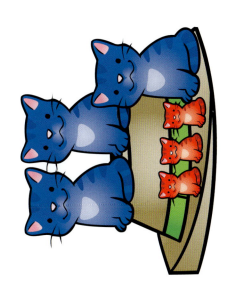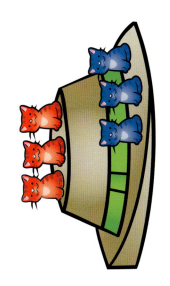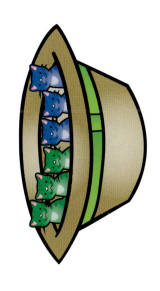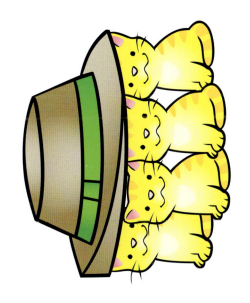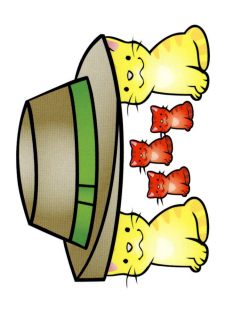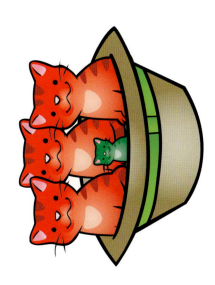

Level 1

Sublevel 30

(+/- quantity + singular/plural) +/- quantity + (size + color + noun) + (prep + pronoun)

Example: Touch the bowl with a few little green balls on it.

1. Touch the only bowl with a few big, red balls on it.

2. Touch the bowl with lots of little, blue balls in it.

3. Touch the bowl with only big, yellow balls in it.

4. Touch the bowl with a few big, yellow balls under it.

5. Touch the bowl with a few little, green balls on it.

6. Touch the only bowl with a big, red ball in it.

©2012 Super Duper® Publications

Plate 4

332

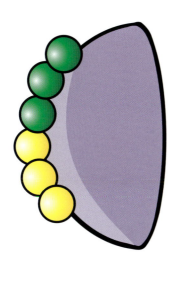
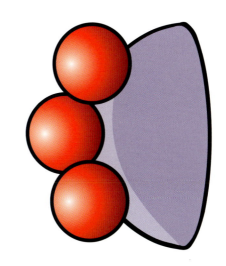
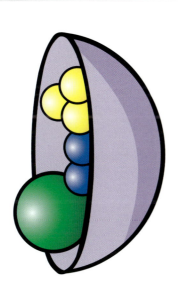
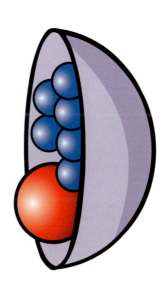
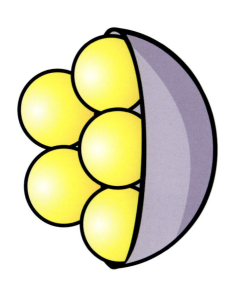
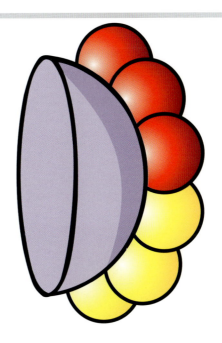

Level 1

Sublevel 30

(+/- quantity + singular/plural) +/- quantity + (size + color + noun) + (prep + pronoun)

Example: Touch the cup with a few big, yellow buttons in it.

1. Touch all the cups with a few little, blue buttons under them.

2. Touch the cup with lots of big, red buttons on it.

3. Touch the only cup with a few little, yellow buttons under it.

4. Touch the cup with only big, red buttons in it.

5. Touch the cup with only little, green buttons under it.

6. Touch the cup with a few big, yellow buttons in it.

©2012 Super Duper® Publications

Plate 5

334

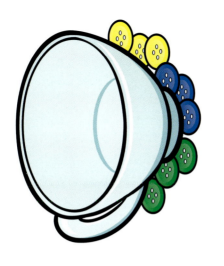
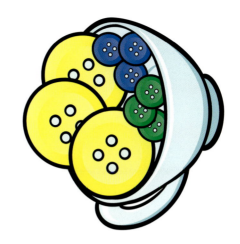
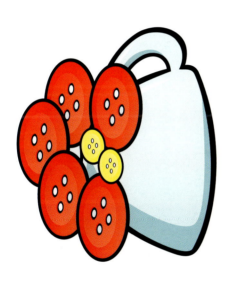
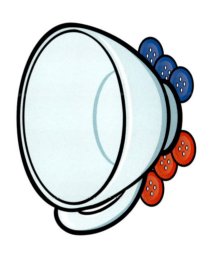
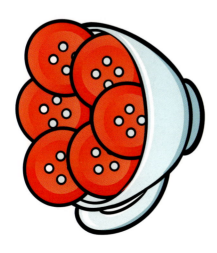
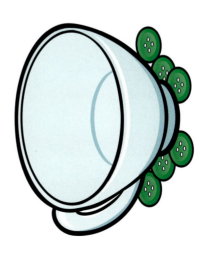

Level 1

Sublevel 31

(+/- quantity + singular/plural) +/- (quantity +/- size + singular/plural) +/- (prep + pronoun)

Example: Touch all the cups with no little beads in them.

1. Touch the cup with only big beads in it.
2. Touch all the cups with no little beads in them.
3. Touch the cup with a few little beads on it.
4. Touch the cup with only one bead under it.
5. Touch the cup with the fewest little beads.

Plate 1

©2012 Super Duper® Publications

336

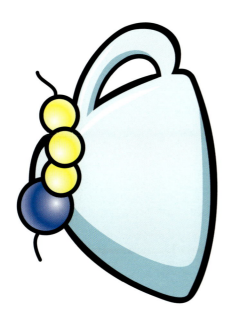
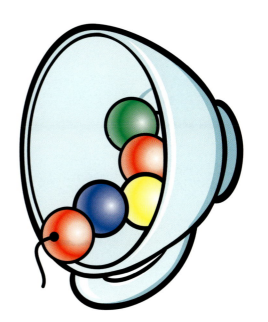
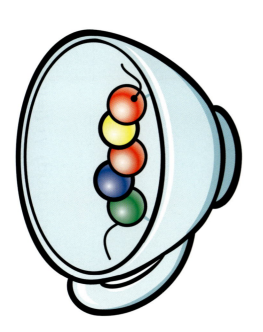
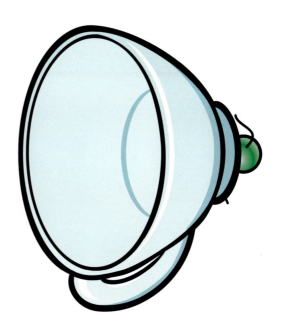

Level 1

Sublevel 31

(+/- quantity + singular/plural) +/- (quantity +/- size + singular/plural) +/- (prep + pronoun)

Example: Touch the cup with only big rings.

1. Touch the cup with a few rings under it.

2. Touch all the cups with no little rings in them.

3. Touch the cup with only big rings.

4. Touch all the cups with one big ring in them.

5. Touch the cup with the most big rings.

©2012 Super Duper® Publications

Plate 2

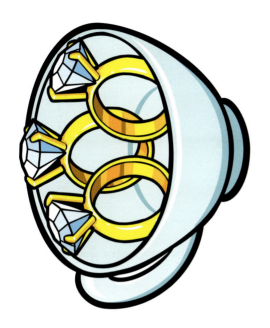
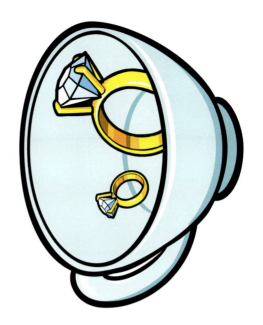
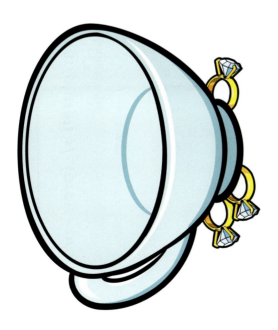
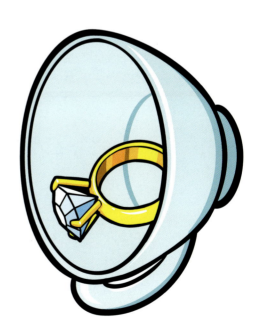

Level 1

Sublevel 31

(+/- quantity + singular/plural) +/- (quantity +/- size + singular/plural) +/- (prep + pronoun)

Example: *Touch the bowl with a few little balls under it.*

1. Touch the bowl with only little balls in it.

2. Touch the only bowl with one little ball.

3. Touch all the bowls with a few big balls in them.

4. Touch the bowl with the most little balls.

5. Touch the bowl with a few little balls under it.

6. Touch the bowl with one big ball under it.

7. Touch the bowl with the fewest little balls.

8. Touch the bowl with some little balls in it.

©2012 Super Duper® Publications

Plate 3

340

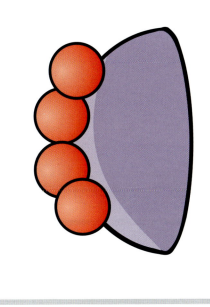
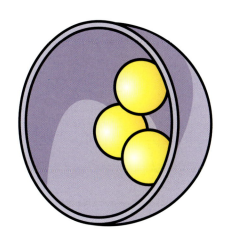
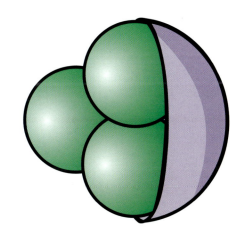
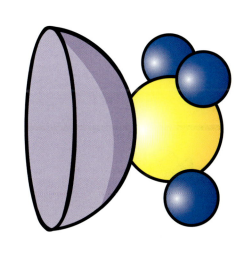
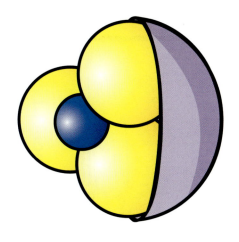
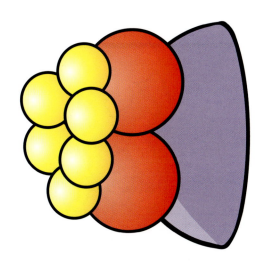

Level 1

Sublevel 31

(+/- quantity + singular/plural) +/- (quantity +/- size + singular/plural) +/- (prep + pronoun)

Example: Touch all the hats with only big frogs.

1. Touch the hat with the most little frogs under it.

2. Touch all the hats with no little frogs.

3. Touch the hat with the most big frogs.

4. Touch the hat with one little frog under it.

5. Touch the hat with the most big frogs in it.

6. Touch all the hats with only big frogs.

7. Touch the hat with the fewest little frogs.

8. Touch all the hats with a few big frogs.

Plate 4

©2012 Super Duper® Publications

342

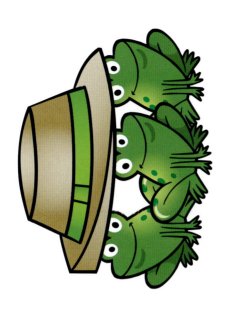
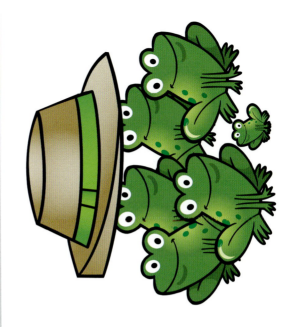
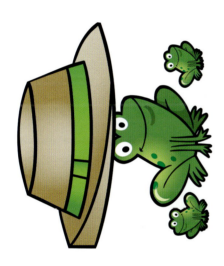
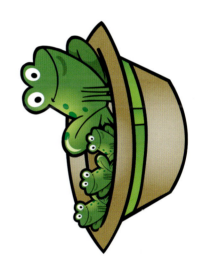
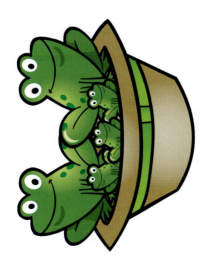
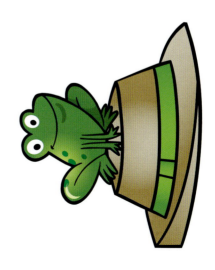

Level 1

Sublevel 31

Plate 5

(+/- **quantity** + **singular/plural**) +/- (**quantity** +/- **size** + **singular/plural**) +/- (**prep** + **pronoun**)

Example: Touch the bowls with only a few big books.

1. Touch the bowl with the most big books on it.

2. Touch the bowl with only a few little books in it.

3. Touch the bowl with the most books under it.

4. Touch the bowl with only a big book.

5. Touch the bowl with lots of little books on it.

6. Touch all the bowls with no little books.

7. Touch the bowl with only little books under it.

8. Touch the bowl with only a little book under it.

9. Touch the bowls with only a few big books.

10. Touch the bowl with the fewest little books.

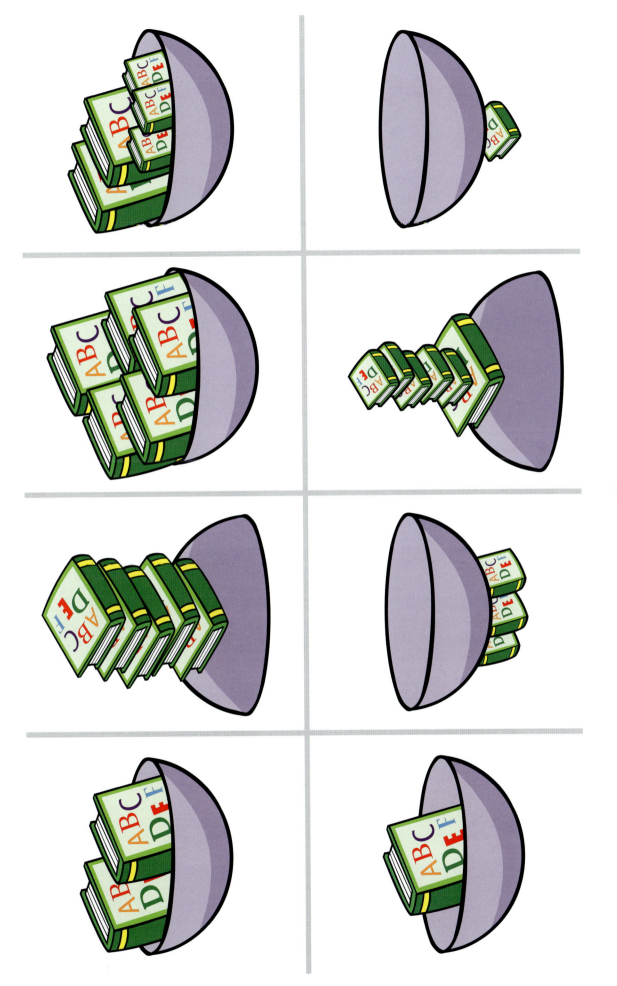

Level 1

Sublevel 31

(+/- quantity + singular/plural) +/- (quantity +/- size + singular/plural) +/- (prep + pronoun)

Example: Touch the cup with a few little buttons in it.

1. Touch the cup with the most big buttons.

2. Touch the only cup with one little button in it.

3. Touch the cup with only little buttons.

4. Touch the cup with only one big button.

5. Touch all the cups with some little buttons.

6. Touch some cups with no buttons in it.

7. Touch the cup with a few little buttons under it.

8. Touch the only cup with one big button in it.

9. Touch the cup with the fewest little buttons.

10. Touch the cup with a few little buttons in it.

Plate 6

©2012 Super Duper® Publications

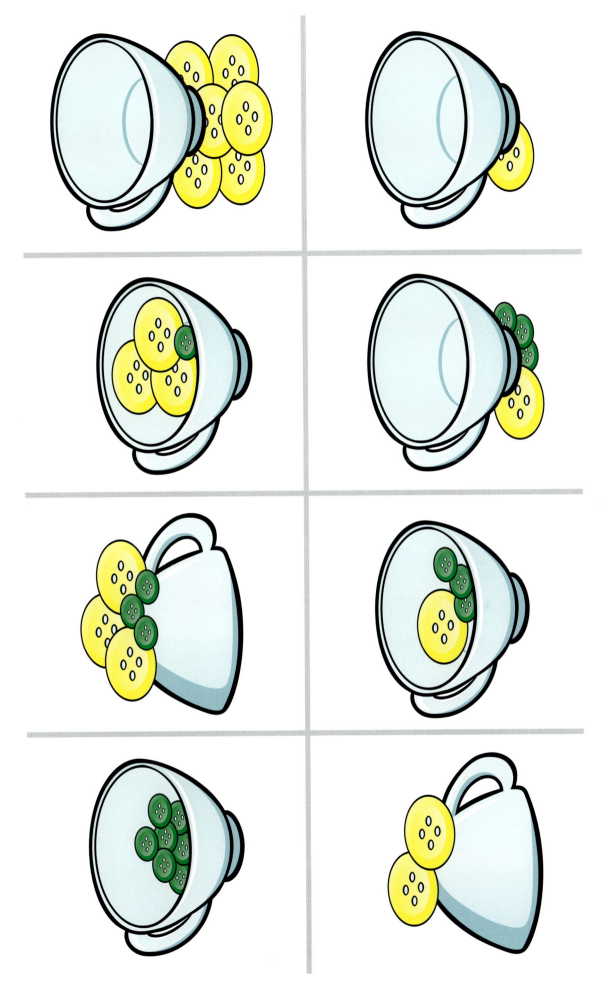

Level 1

Sublevel 32

(+/- quantity + singular/plural) +/- (quantity +/- size +/- color + singular/plural) +/- (prep + pronoun)

Example: Touch the cup a lot of little, red beads.

1. Touch all the cups with some little beads on them.

2. Touch the cup a lot of little, red beads.

3. Touch the only cup with one big bead in it.

4. Touch the cup with the most big, blue beads.

5. Touch the cup with a few little, green beads in it.

6. Touch all the cups with no beads in them.

©2012 Super Duper® Publications

Plate 1

348

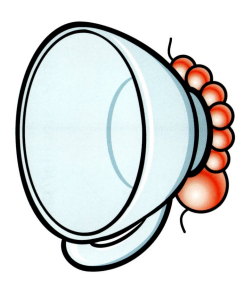
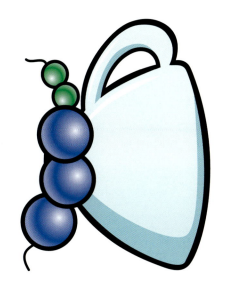
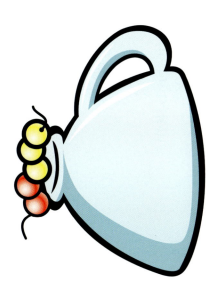
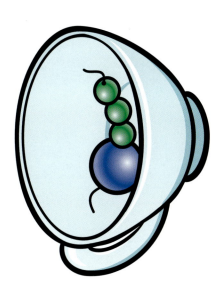

Level 1

Sublevel 32

(+/- quantity + singular/plural) +/- (quantity +/- size + color + singular/plural) +/- (prep + pronoun)

Example: Touch all the bowls with a few big balls in them.

1. Touch the bowl with the most little, green balls.

2. Touch the bowl with only a little ball under it.

3. Touch all the bowls with a few big balls in them.

4. Touch the bowl with a few little balls on it.

5. Touch the bowl with only one big ball on it.

6. Touch all the bowls with no balls in them.

Plate 2

©2012 Super Duper® Publications

350

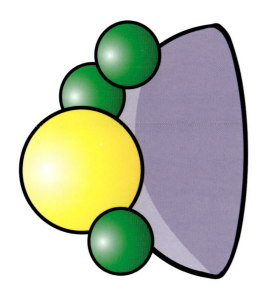
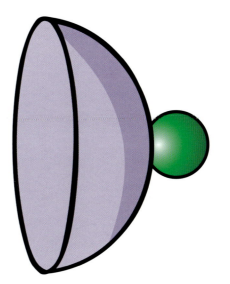
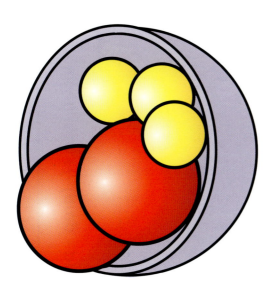
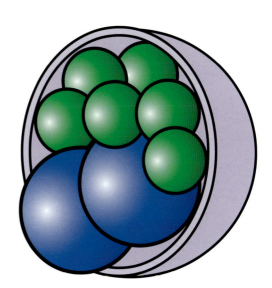

Level 1

Sublevel 32

(+/- **quantity** + **singular/plural**) +/- (**quantity** +/- **size** +/- **color** + **singular/plural**) +/- (**prep** + **pronoun**)

Example: *Touch the hat with the most cats on it.*

1. Touch the hat with a few big, yellow cats.

2. Touch the only hat with some red cats in it.

3. Touch the only hat with one big cat under it.

4. Touch the hat with a few big, blue cats.

5. Touch the hat with the most cats on it.

6. Touch some of the hats with no cats on them.

7. Touch all the hats with some little, blue cats.

8. Touch the hat with the fewest little, blue cats.

©2012 Super Duper® Publications

Plate 3

352

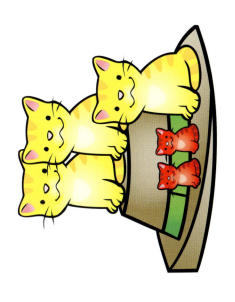
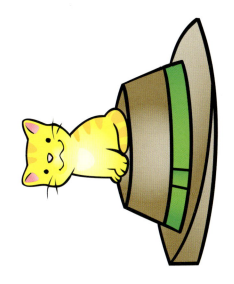
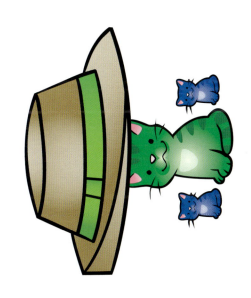
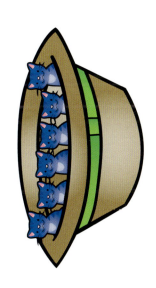
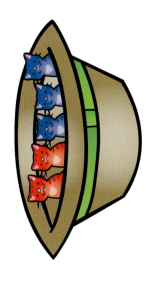
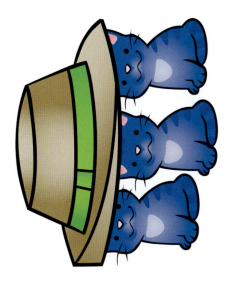

Level 1

Sublevel 32

(+/- **quantity** + **singular/plural**) **+/-** (**quantity** +/- **size** +/- **color** + **singular/plural**) **+/-** (**prep** + **pronoun**)

Example: Touch the only bowl with some big, yellow shoes.

1. Touch the bowl with the most little, yellow shoes.
2. Touch some bowls with no red shoes under them.
3. Touch the only bowl with a few little, blue shoes.
4. Touch the bowl with the fewest shoes under it.
5. Touch the bowl with a few big shoes in it.
6. Touch the only bowl with some big, yellow shoes.
7. Touch all the bowls with no shoes in them.
8. Touch the bowl with the most little, blue shoes.

©2012 Super Duper® Publications

Plate 4

354

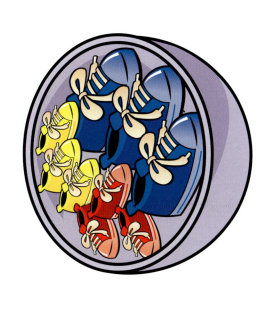
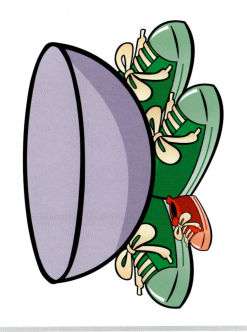
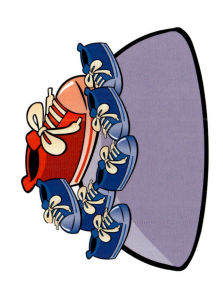
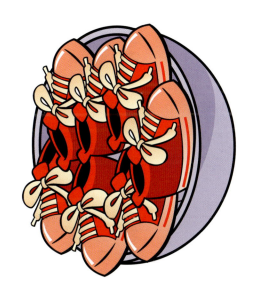
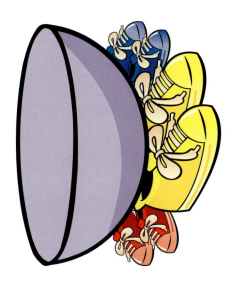
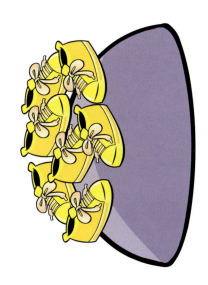

32-4

Level 1

Sublevel 32

(+/- quantity + singular/plural) +/- (quantity +/- size +/- color + singular/plural) +/- (prep + pronoun)

Example: *Touch the hat with the fewest little, red dogs.*

1. Touch the hat with the most big, blue dogs.
2. Touch the hat with a few little, red dogs in it.
3. Touch the hat with a few little, blue dogs on it.
4. Touch the hat with only one, big dog on it.
5. Touch all the hats with some little dogs in them.
6. Touch the hat with a few big, green dogs in it.
7. Touch the hat with the most little, yellow dogs.
8. Touch the hat with only red dogs under it.
9. Touch the hat with the fewest little, red dogs.
10. Touch the hat with only a few big, red dogs.

Plate 5

©2012 Super Duper® Publications

356

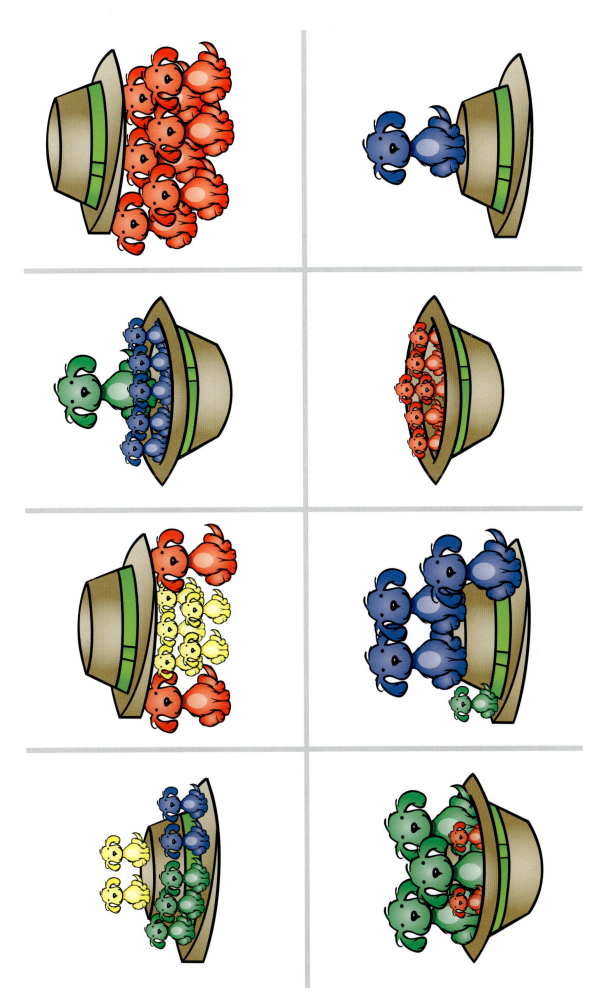

Level 1

Sublevel 32

(+/- quantity + singular/plural) +/- (quantity +/- size +/- color + singular/plural) +/- (prep + pronoun)

Example: Touch all the cups with no buttons in them.

1. Touch the cup with the most little, yellow buttons under it.

2. Touch the cup with a few big, yellow buttons in it.

3. Touch all the cups with no yellow buttons.

4. Touch the cup with lots of little, green buttons on it.

5. Touch the cup with the most little, red buttons.

6. Touch the cup with the fewest yellow buttons in it.

7. Touch the only cup with one big button on it.

8. Touch the cup with the most blue buttons in it.

9. Touch the cup with the fewest little, green buttons.

10. Touch all the cups with no buttons in them.

©2012 Super Duper® Publications

Plate 6

358

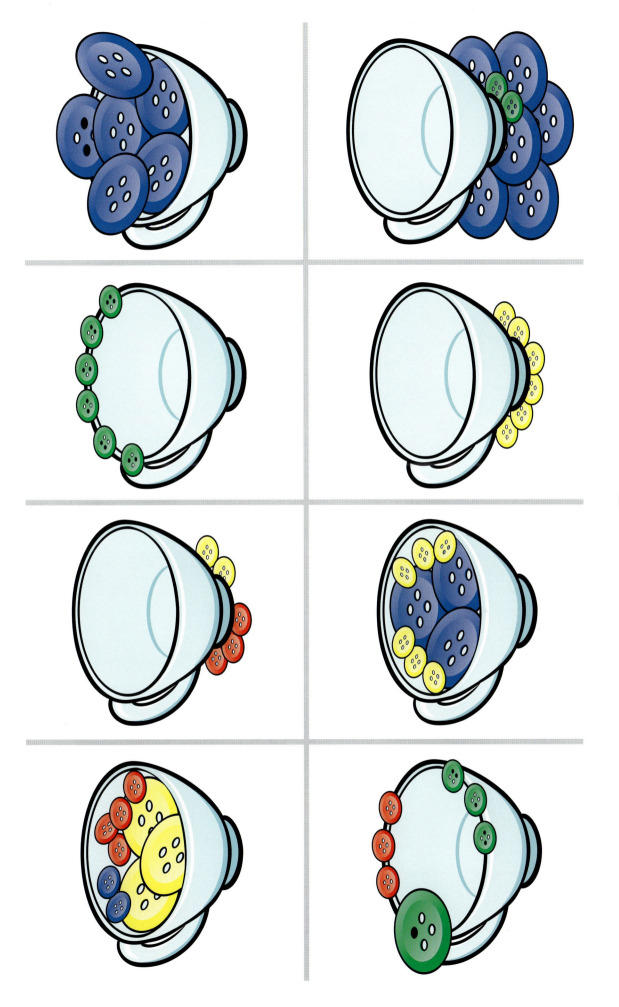